Ask CosmoGIRL!

About Nutrition and Fitness

From the Editors of CosmoGIRL!

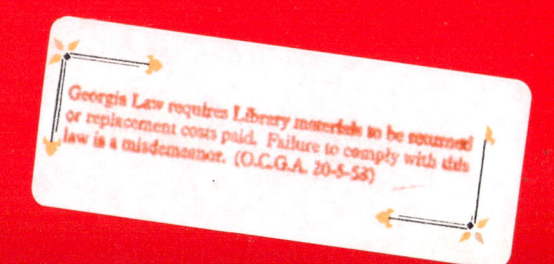

Ask COSMOgirl!

About Nutrition and Fitness

From the Editors of CosmoGIRL!

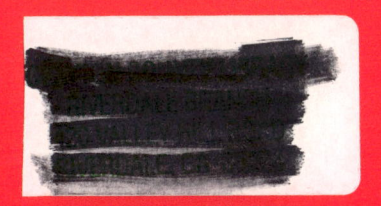

HEARST BOOKS
A division of Sterling Publishing Co., Inc.

New York / London
www.sterlingpublishing.com

Copyright © 2008 by Hearst Communications, Inc.

All rights reserved.

Library of Congress Cataloging-in-Publication Data

Ask Cosmogirl! about nutrition and fitness / from the editors of Cosmogirl!
     p. cm.
  Includes index.
  ISBN-13: 978-1-58816-645-6
  ISBN-10: 1-58816-645-7
 1. Teenage girls–Nutrition. 2. Young women–Nutrition. 3. Teenage girls–Health and hygiene. 4. Young women–Health and hygiene. 5. Weight loss. I. Cosmo girl.
  RJ235.A85 2007
  613'.04243–dc22

2007001670

10 9 8 7 6 5 4 3 2

Published by Hearst Books
A Division of Sterling Publishing Co., Inc.
387 Park Avenue South, New York, NY 10016

CosmoGIRL! and Hearst Books are trademarks of Hearst Communications, Inc.

www.cosmogirl.com

For information about custom editions, special sales, premium and corporate purchases, please contact Sterling Special Sales Department at 800-805-5489 or specialsales@sterlingpub.com.

Distributed in Canada by Sterling Publishing
c/o Canadian Manda Group, 165 Dufferin Street
Toronto, Ontario, Canada M6K 3H6

Distributed in Australia by Capricorn Link (Australia) Pty. Ltd.
P.O. Box 704, Windsor, NSW 2756 Australia

Manufactured in China

Sterling ISBN 13: 978-1-58816-645-6
        ISBN 10: 1-58816-645-7

Photography Credits: Page 10 Nino Muñoz Page 72 Dominique Palombo Page 94 Nino Muñoz Page 112 Nino Muñoz

contents

Foreword
Susan's Note: A letter from our Editor-in-Chief 8

Chapter 1: A Healthy Diet 10

Chapter 2: Work it Out 72

Chapter 3: Love Your Body 94

Chapter 4: Weighty Issues 112

Index 124

foreword

Hey CosmoGIRL!s,

Want to know something that used to surprise me as the editor of your favorite magazine? The great response we get from you about our fitness and nutrition stories! I guess I used to think that you might see fitness and nutrition as homework—as opposed to something fun. But from the thousands of emails I get from you, I've learned that you're **very** interested in and motivated about taking care of yourselves. And that makes me **really** happy. You never hesitate to ask about healthy food options or good exercise moves that will give you more energy to do all the cool things you do in your life. And with so many headlines screaming out about either eating disorders or obesity, it makes sense that you'd want to take charge of your body's health. It's just one more way that you impress me by being so smart and put-together.

This book is packed with tons of questions you've asked us. You can use it as a resource whenever you're wondering about something, or just read it to see what other girls are asking about, so you know that whatever your fitness or nutrition dilemma, you're not alone. Keep your questions coming to me at **susan@cosmogirl.com**. I'm here to listen and you just might see your question answered in the magazine!

Until then… may you use this book in good health!

Love,

Susan

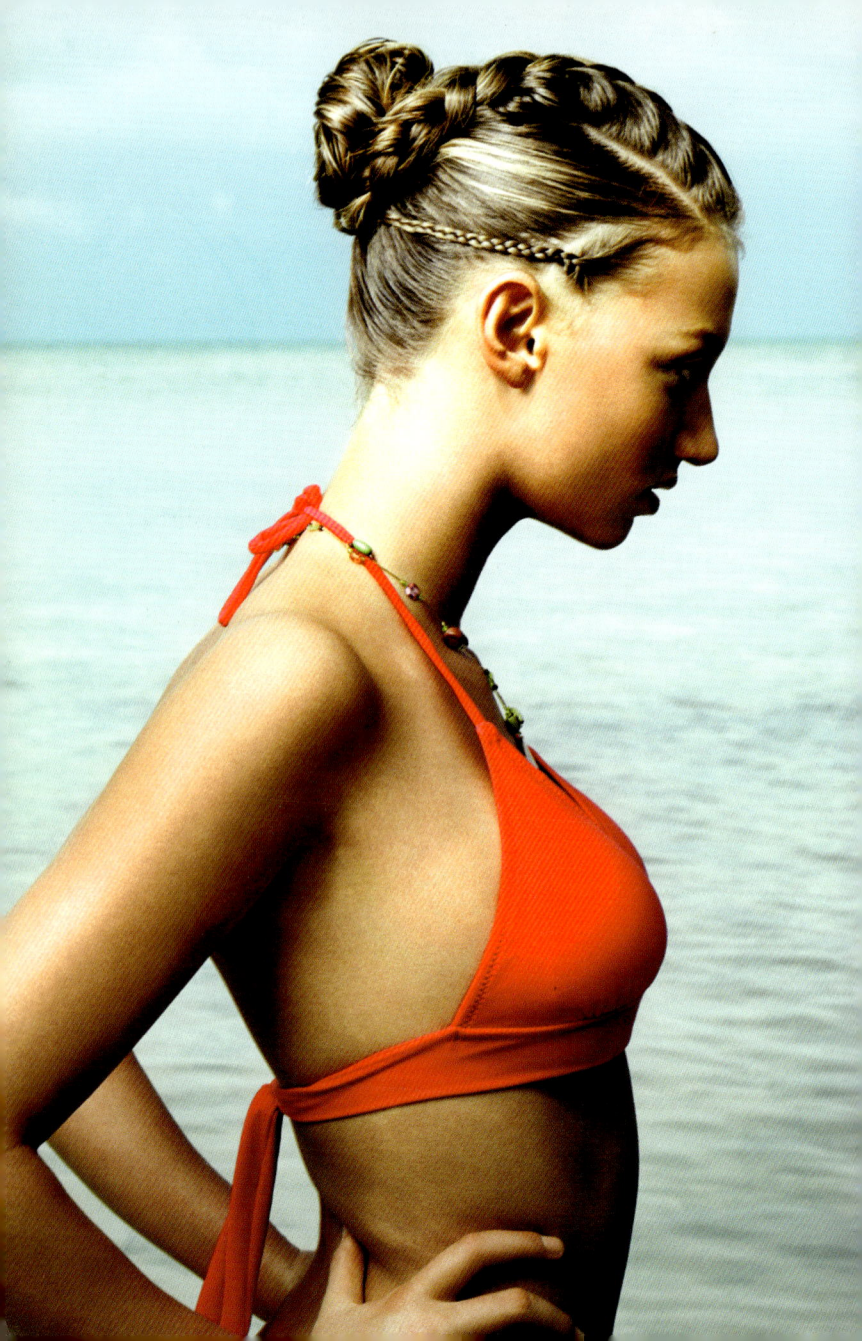

chapter 1

a healthy diet

Maintaining a healthy weight means having a healthy diet, but listen up CosmoGIRL!s: It doesn't mean actually being on a diet! Diet means what you do eat—not what you don't. Find out some of the questions your fellow CG!s have asked about how to eat healthfully, and use our advice to get fit!

a healthy diet

Q **I want to establish healthy eating habits for myself, but with all the information out there, I can't make sense of what I should be doing. Help!**

A You have enough to worry about with school, friends, and family. Why is eating, something we do to survive, so anxiety-inducing? Eating should energize you, not stress you out! So we'll cut through all the chaos and get to the honest truth about eating healthfully.

- *First, respect your body.* Metabolisms vary from person to person, which means you should focus on your metabolism and not your friends'. When you know how your body works, it will be much easier to give it what it needs.
- *Next, change your vocabulary when it comes to food.* Eating isn't a film with good guys and bad guys. When you say things like "I was good today" when you skip dessert or "I was bad" because you had ice cream, you train yourself to feel guilty about food. Instead, refer to foods like fruit and veggies as "everyday" foods, and cake and chips as "sometimes" foods.
- *Be sure to savor your food.* When you sit down to a meal, really focus on your food. Slowly chew each bite and think

about how it tastes and feels. You'll enjoy your food more and appreciate how it refuels your body. Plus, if you slow down, you'll end up feeling full after eating the perfect satisfying amount.

- *Don't skip meals.* Skipping meals won't make you thin; it will make your body think it's starving and, as a result, your metabolism will slow down. Eat three nutritious meals and two snacks a day for an efficient metabolism.
- *Pick healthy carbs.* "Carb" has become a four-letter word thanks to some fad diets. But complex carbohydrates keep your blood sugar level up so you stay energized, plus they provide you with healthy fiber. So choose fruits and whole grains like nutrient-rich, whole-wheat bread or pasta instead of empty carbs like white bread or white rice.
- *Don't forget to indulge yourself once in a while.* Of course you'll get cravings for chips or cookies—who doesn't? When you do, treat yourself to a small portion. Give your body what it's asking for and you'll satisfy the urge. Deny yourself and eventually you'll break down and eat a ton of junk! Make all this information second nature, and the word "diet" will mean *what* you eat—not what you don't!

a healthy diet

breakfast matters

Q: I skip breakfast so I can lose weight, but it doesn't seem to be working. If I cut the extra calories, why won't the pounds drop off?

A: We know you've heard this before: Breakfast is the most important meal of the day. The one thing we can say about clichés is that if they get used so much, perhaps there's some truth to them. It comes down to this: You've got to eat breakfast. If you don't, your metabolism doesn't get its daily jump start—so then when you eat later, your body doesn't burn calories as efficiently. Also, skipping breakfast may cause you to eat more at lunch and dinner or snack at night because you're hungry. Think about it: Skipping breakfast could actually make you gain weight!

Q: I'm just not hungry in the morning. Should I force myself to eat, even if if makes me want to puke?

A: Whoa—no puking, please! Just because you have to start eating breakfast doesn't mean you need to gobble up a "trucker's special" of eggs, bacon, sausage, toast, pancakes, etc., your first morning. Work up to it. You need to train your body to develop a morning appetite, not force it to digest all kinds of things. Start by having a glass of skim milk or a latte made with skim milk every morning for a week. The next week, add a piece of fruit. By the third week, you'll probably notice that you're hungrier in the mornings, and then you can aim for a 300- to 400-calorie breakfast with complex carbs, protein, and fiber.

CG! TIP: If you need an AM jump start, choose coffee rather than soda. It has antioxidants, which may help keep your heart healthy and your skin looking young.

a healthy diet

Q: Why do I feel so tired after eating breakfast?

A A morning meal with too much sugar could be the cause of your post-breakfast slump. And lots of products that don't necessarily taste sweet still contain simple sugars—for example, juice, cereal bars, muffins, and bread. For energy boosters that won't make you crash, try a breakfast of carbs, protein, and fiber. Eat an orange (fiber), bran muffin (complex carbs and fiber), and skim milk (protein), or go for whole-wheat toast (complex carbs and fiber) and peanut butter (protein) instead of buttered white toast. A third option? Have a sugary cereal bar, but pair it with a light yogurt (protein) and an apple (complex carbs).

Q: I need a quick solution for a healthy breakfast. Any suggestions?

A Try a tropical smoothie. It's high in fiber and packed with antioxidants and protein, which help you stay energized all day. And it's really quick and easy to make! Combine 1 kiwi, peeled and cut into ¼ inch chunks, half a mango, peeled and cut into ¼-inch chunks, 1 cup orange juice, 2 cups apple juice, 1 cup extra-firm light tofu (in the produce section) in a blender and blend on high until smooth (about 30 seconds). Pour into a glass and drink up!

Q: I get so sluggish by the end of second period. What can I eat that won't make me crash?

A: Try an egg white scramble and a smoothie. Here's what you need for the scramble: 1 slice of multigrain bread, 2 egg whites, 1 tablespoon. Dijon mustard, and salt and pepper to taste. Preheat a small skillet and pop the bread into the toaster. Separate the egg whites by cracking eggs over a bowl and tossing the yolks between the shell halves until all of the whites drop into the bowl. Discard the yolks. Coat the skillet with cooking spray and mix the whites around with a spatula until fully cooked (about 2–5 minutes). Spread mustard on the toasted bread and top with eggs for an open-faced sandwich. Add salt and pepper. For the smoothie, place one banana, 2 cups strawberries, and ½ cup soy milk in a blender and blend for about a minute. Then, drink up—yum!

a healthy diet

Q I've totally cut fat out of what I eat in the morning, but now I start getting hungry even an hour after I eat. Can you recommend any nonfattening and filling foods I can eat in the morning without worrying about packing on the pounds?

A We've got to let you in on something here: Having no fat in your diet, especially at breakfast, is actually not a great thing. It's important to eat a well-balanced breakfast with fat to help you feel full, protein to help your muscles recover, and carbs to give you energy. That doesn't mean bacon or sausage, though. There are other options. Try making a smoothie with 1 cup soy milk, 1 cup strawberries, and 2 tablespoons ground flaxseed (available at health-food stores), which has fiber and the good kind of fat.

party tricks

Q **I'm going to my cousin's wedding next month, and I'm really afraid of overeating. I've been on a diet now for several weeks and I've been doing well, but how can I control myself with all the delicious food they'll have there?**

A Don't worry. You can have a great time at the wedding, sample a whole bunch of the savory selections—and not kill all the progress you've made. Just follow these guidelines. First, don't eat directly from serving bowls or plates. When grazing during the cocktail reception, place food on a plate. This will help you better judge how much you're eating. Be sure to survey the entire food spread before digging in. You might be sorry you already ate a meatball when you find your favorite pasta on the other side of the room! Finally, skip the hot mini pastries or fried appetizers that get passed around. Usually the offerings from the buffet table, like veggies and dip, cheese and crackers, and sushi, are much healthier—and easier to track. And remember: A wedding may be a great opportunity to overeat, but it also features a built-in way to work off that food. Get up on the dance floor at the reception and shake your booty!

CG! TIP: Make sure you're eating at least a cup of fruits and vegetables at every meal!

a healthy diet

Q **I want to have some friends over and I'm looking for some healthy, tasty snack suggestions. Any ideas?**

A If healthy is what you crave, you definitely want to stay away from finger foods like pigs in a blanket, which have lots of salt and fat. These Asian wraps are a great alternative. Instead of bread and mini hot dogs, they are made from warm chicken flavored with herbs and a low-fat sauce, wrapped in cool, crisp lettuce leaves. And they're delish! Here's what you need to make about 16 wraps: Canola oil cooking spray, 1 pound ground chicken breast, 1 tablespoon black bean sauce, 1 tablespoon water, 6 shiitake mushrooms (chopped, stems removed) 2 tablespoons chopped chives, and 8 leaves iceberg lettuce, torn into 3-by-3-inch pieces. First, coat a sauté pan with cooking spray. Add the chicken and cook until browned, stirring to break up the meat (about 8 minutes). Mix black bean sauce with water, then add the mixture to the chicken. Stir until blended and remove from heat. To make each wrap, place large spoonfuls of chicken mixture on a lettuce piece, roll lengthwise, and pierce with a toothpick.

Q **I need a low-fat alternative to the dip my mom usually makes for veggies. Any suggestions for one that's healthy—but still yummy?**

A Lots of dips are made with fattening mayonnaise, but this tzatziki dip calls for nonfat yogurt, which makes the dip tangy and creamy and is a great source of protein and calcium. To make enough for a group of about 12 to 16, you'll need: 2 medium cucumbers, 4 teaspoons salt, 2 cups plain nonfat yogurt, 4 cloves garlic (minced) 1 tablespoon chopped fresh mint, 1 tablespoon chopped fresh dill, and 4 teaspoons lemon juice. For dipping, you'll also need 6 whole-wheat pitas, plus celery and carrot sticks. To make: Peel cucumbers, slice them lengthwise, scoop out the seeds and discard, then grate cucumbers with a cheese grater. Put grated cucumbers in a clean paper towel and squeeze out as much moisture as you can over the sink. Place cucumbers in a bowl and mix in salt. Refrigerate mixture for an hour. Remove cucumbers from fridge and stir in remaining ingredients. Refrigerate mixture for 2 hours, then serve with pita triangles and sliced vegetables.

a healthy diet

Q: My friends and I are planning a girls' movie night. What can we snack on that's not greasy and salty—but still good to eat?

A: How about fruit salsa with pita chips? To make enough for four people, you'll need: 4 whole-wheat pita pockets, ¼ cup olive oil, 1 cup diced mango or papaya, 1 cup diced pineapple, 2 tablespoons chopped cilantro, ¼ cup diced onion, 2 tablespoons honey, 1 tablespoon lime juice. Preheat oven to 425 degrees. Cut pitas into 8 triangles and brush tops with oil. Place pita pieces on a baking sheet, oil side up, and bake for 10 minutes. While the pita is baking, make salsa by combining the remaining ingredients in a medium bowl. Serve fruit salsa with pita chips. Just half a cup of this salsa counts as one of your daily fruit servings (you need three a day), and the whole-wheat pita chips are healthier than potato or tortilla chips!

Q: It's my boyfriend's birthday and I want to make him dinner. He loves Tex-Mex food, but it seems so fattening to me. Is there something I can make for him that will make both of us happy?

A: We have the perfect recipe! These roasted veggie quesadillas have Tex-Mex flavor and lots of gooey cheese, but they've also got two servings of vegetables (you need at least four a day), and less fat than most Mexican food. And they're pretty easy! First, preheat the oven to 450 degrees. Dice ¼ cup zucchini, ¼ cup red bell pepper, ¼ cup green bell pepper, and ¼ cup onion. Toss in a bowl with ½ teaspoon chili powder. Spread mixture over a baking sheet and drizzle with 1 tablespoon olive oil, and bake 10 minutes or until veggies are tender. Then, place two 12-inch whole-wheat tortillas in skillet. Cook 2 minutes, flip, then spread with veggie mixture and ⅓ cup shredded low-fat Monterey Jack cheese, and cook until cheese melts. Remove from heat, cut into quarters, and enjoy!

a healthy diet

season's eating

Q: Help! Every year at the holidays, my Italian family makes a ton of food and it's all so good, I can't control myself. I don't want to plump up like Santa this Christmas—but how can I enjoy myself while everyone around me's digging in?

A: It may be easier than you think. First of all, don't eat everything in sight. Eat smart and you can still enjoy yourself. One tip is to pick the darker food: red sauce instead of creamy, sweet potatoes rather than white, spinach instead of lettuce. Usually the deeper the color of a food, the healthier it is. Also, you know how family and friends like to schmooze before sitting down for the big feast? Have a few sticks of celery topped with peanut butter as a pre-party snack—it will keep you from gorging when the first course is finally served. If you have the opportunity to bring a food to the event, make the best of it. Low-fat tortilla chips with salsa or air-popped popcorn sprayed with butter-flavored cooking spray and sprinkled with cinnamon sugar taste just as good as junk food. Last but far from least, don't skip other meals beforehand! Eating breakfast and lunch will satisfy you and actually prevent you from overeating later in the day!

dining out

Q: I heard that people who eat out a lot have more of a chance of getting fat than people who eat together at home. Is this really true?

A: Scientifically speaking, yes. Studies have shown that teens who eat dinner at home with their families have healthier diets, but of course that depends on how well you eat at home. If you're all standing over the stove, picking at the heated frozen fries someone remembered to take out of the oven, and supplementing with snacks from the fridge, that's not gonna cut it. You have to change that! How? Suggest to your parents that you eat together as a family at least three times a week and try to build up to five if your schedules allow. Take the initiative of putting together one or more of these meals yourself—and make them healthy! And if your family's short on time in the evenings, make it a breakfast dinner of scrambled eggs, toast, and fruit salad.

CG! TIP: Find healthy family recipes at www.teenshealth.org.

a healthy diet

Q: My family and I eat out a lot. Do you have any tips for healthy menu selections?

A: Choose grilled or baked items rather than fried or sautéed ones—requesting an item "grilled dry" (without oil) is even better. Look for menu options that are cooked with Cajun seasoning or herbs—they'll be just as flavorful. Always order condiments on the side so you can control how much of them you eat. Finally, restaurant portions are usually huge. Eat half your meal, then have the other half wrapped up—lunch the next day—so you won't overindulge. If you're not into leftovers, we bet your dad or brother will be happy to finish it for you!

Q **What's better for you: an egg and cheese on an English muffin, a smoothie, or a reduced-fat blueberry muffin?**

A You're not going to believe us, but, in this case, the egg sandwich wins! It has more protein than the smoothie and less fat than the muffin. Shocked? Well, it's true. You might as well call that muffin a cupcake because it has 12 grams of fat (the regular muffin has 17 grams), lots of sugar, and little protein (which gives you energy and helps you feel full longer). The smoothie is better, but it has little protein, and though it's a drink, because it's made from fruit, it contains tons of sugar.

CG! Tip: Look for the percentage of trans fat, now listed on labels. These hydrogenated or partially hydrogenated oils are processed in a lab and unhealthy—avoid them at all costs!

a healthy diet

Q **My friends and I like to chow down on fast food sometimes, but we'd still like to try to be healthy when we do. Any suggestions on what we should order?**

A Surprise! A burger and small fries has less fat than some other options, and if you add a side salad, you'll get fiber and essential vitamins and minerals. With fat-free dressing on the salad, assume 24 grams of fat. Other popular choices are a toss-up: A grilled chicken salad with fat-free dressing and fries can have 31 grams of fat; a typical burrito can have up to 33 grams of fat. And remember, when you order a salad, all the add-ons can make it less healthy than you think. When you order, ask them to hold the cheese, croutons, and any other non-vegetable or fruit topping—and get your dressing on the side.

Q **When I eat out, I always order a salad to be healthy, and then French fries so I can feel satisfied without eating any fattening meat. But I usually get hungry again in an hour or so. Why?**

A The problem here is that while you may feel full right after you eat this combo, it lacks protein and dairy, so it's technically not a complete meal, and therefore, won't carry you through. Plus, fries have tons of fat, and restaurants usually use iceberg lettuce, which has about the same nutritional value as water (none!). Instead of your usual, why not try ordering a baked potato and a spinach salad with colorful veggies like tomatoes and carrots. For protein, have milk instead of soda, or try a fruit and yogurt parfait for dessert. Or go for a veggie pizza (there's protein in the cheese)!

a healthy diet

Q **My friend wants to celebrate her sixteenth birthday at a restaurant. I've been on a diet, so I downloaded the menu to see if there was anything offered that I could get away with eating. What's better: fried chicken salad, an appetizer or two, or chicken fajitas?**

A In this situation, the chicken fajitas are the best choice. Many restaurants have low-carb options, but most experts agree that low-carb diets aren't healthy for teens. And just because something is an appetizer doesn't mean it is smaller or has fewer calories than an entrée. Salads (like ones topped with fried chicken, cheese, and creamy dressing) can have more fat and calories than an entrée!

metabolism 411

Q: What's the deal with this thing called metabolism, and what does it have to do with losing weight?

A: Metabolism is the process your body goes through to turn calories into energy. But metabolism isn't the only thing that determines weight; it's how much you eat and exercise that matters. Exercising does increase your metabolism, both while and after you work out. If you exercise enough to build more muscle, your resting metabolic rate (the speed of your metabolism when you're doing nothing) will be higher too. That's because muscle cells use energy (to create motion for everything from your heart beating to your mouth smiling); fat cells just sit there. Your metabolism is slowest when you're sleeping and fastest when you're exercising. That's why breakfast is important—eating in the morning tells your body that it's time to start burning calories. If you don't eat, your metabolism will still operate in night mode (slowly!).

a healthy diet

Q: Do skinny people always have fast metabolisms and larger people have slow ones?

A: Skinny people don't always have faster metabolisms. Actually, overweight people do. Surprised? Think about it. It takes more energy to operate something bigger, so bigger people use more energy to do the same things smaller people do. When you skip meals, your body thinks it's starving, so it slows down your metabolism to make the calories you do take in last longer. If you want to lose weight, keep your metabolism steady by choosing foods with fewer calories (pretzels instead of chips, for example) rather than eating less or skipping meals. You can't boost your metabolism with an energy drink. Energy drinks usually have caffeine, which can slightly speed up your heart rate. When that happens, your metabolism increases temporarily, but that temporary boost doesn't burn enough calories for you to actually lose weight.

don't ditch dessert!

Q: My best friend's birthday is coming up this weekend, and I'm looking for a healthy substitute for cake to make for her. Any ideas?

A A mixed-berry trifle is sweet and creamy—and virtually fat-free. Plus, the berries are a great source of antioxidants and vitamins. It's also pretty simple. Here's what you need to make this tasty treat for a group of 12 to 16: One 8- or 9-inch angel food cake, a 5-ounce box of fat-free vanilla instant pudding mix, 3 cups nonfat milk, a 12-ounce container of fat-free whipped topping, three 12-ounce packages frozen mixed berries (keep frozen), and 1 cup fresh berries for garnish. To put it together, cut the cake into 1-inch cubes; set aside. In a large bowl, mix the pudding mix and milk. Reserve 1 cup whipped topping, then fold in remaining topping. Put half the cake pieces and half the frozen berries in a large trifle bowl (or any large glass bowl); top with half the pudding mixture. Repeat the layering process once more. Garnish with reserved whipped topping and fresh berries. Cover and chill 3 to 4 hours before serving, and voilà!

a healthy diet

Q **I love to have something sweet after dinner, and I usually pig out on ice cream. That's probably why I can't fit in to any of my cool jeans anymore! Can you suggest an alternative that's just as tasty—without all the fat and calories in ice cream?**

A A strawberry-yogurt parfait is cool and refreshing like ice cream, but it has much less fat and sugar. Plus, the yogurt counts as one serving of dairy (you need at least three a day). Here's how to make it. In a bowl, toss together ¾ cup sliced strawberries, 1 teaspoon honey, and ½ teaspoon chopped fresh rosemary or mint. Into a clear glass, spoon 3 ounces (roughly half a container) of low-fat vanilla yogurt, and top with berry mixture. Finish with a yogurt layer, then garnish with a sprig of mint or rosemary, and eat up!

Q **My sister got a fondue set for Christmas, and it's so much fun, we use it just about every night! Any healthier suggestions than the standard melted chocolate or cheese?**

A This chocolate chip fondue dip is made with prunes (they add fiber and sweetness) and fat-free milk instead of cream, so it's low-fat. Plus, it contains calcium and protein. Combine 1 cup semisweet chocolate chips and ½ cup fat-free evaporated milk in a fondue pot. Heat mixture over low heat, stirring constantly until smooth (about 5 minutes). Slowly add a 2.5-ounce jar of baby food prunes, stirring until blended. Use strawberries, apple slices, and graham crackers as dippers.

a healthy diet

you are what you drink

Q **I've always heard you should avoid coffee if you want to stay healthy, but lately I've been hearing that coffee's good for you. Am I going nuts? What's the deal?**

A No, you're not going nuts. A cup o' joe can actually be good for you! Coffee has gotten a bad rap, but research shows there are some good things about the buzzy brew. The caffeine can help you with complex brain functions, like figuring out math problems. And some studies show that coffee may also help to keep your liver healthy. But high-calorie coffee concoctions like full-fat lattes or mochaccinos? Not so much. With 300 calories or more, they can have as many calories as a meal but they don't fill you up! So go ahead and drink coffee—just don't overdo it.

Q: Which is better for you, iced or warm coffee—and why?

A It's not the temperature of the coffee that's the issue, it's what gets added to it. Many cold coffee drinks are made from sugary mixes or even ice cream, so if you do reach for a cold one, go for plain iced coffee or an iced latte with skim milk and add your own sweetener. It's healthier than a thick, smoothie-like coffee drink. But coffee should never be used as a meal substitute. For one, chewing helps your body register fullness, so having a 300-calorie iced coffee drink won't fill you up like a 300-calorie meal.

CG! TIP: Go easy on the 'cino: A tall Starbucks Frappuccino has 190 calories and 20 grams of fat, but a Venti has 350 calories and 40 grams of fat!

a healthy diet

Q: I've heard the caffeine in coffee is really good for helping you lose weight. Is this true?

A: Yes and no. Caffeine can lead to weight loss as it stimulates the body and enhances fat metabolism. It's also a diuretic, so that means less bloating. That's why many of those weight-loss, "fat-burner" supplements you see on the shelves actually contain caffeine. But there are drawbacks. The moisture you lose from the diuretic effect can lead to dehydration, constipation, headaches, and there are other side effects with caffeine, including sleeplessness and irritability. Caffeine can also trigger weight gain. It induces stress in the body, which sparks the production of cortisol, a stress hormone that in large amounts leads to the accumulation of belly fat.

Q: How much water should I be drinking every day?

A: You *might* need 8 glasses to stay hydrated; it depends on how active you are, your body size, and your environment. You're hydrated when your pee is pale yellow and you aren't thirsty (thirst is a sign of dehydration). Think of water as your energy elixir. Staying hydrated helps prevent fatigue. Plus, you'll be less likely to reach for a soda or candy.

Q: What's better for you after a workout: a sugar-free energy drink, a bottle of water, or a half-pint of chocolate milk?

A: After a workout that lasts more than an hour, chocolate milk is better than water or caffeine-loaded energy drinks like Red Bull. Milk has carbs, which aid in rehydration and provide fuel for muscles, plus protein, which helps muscles recover more quickly. But if you work out for less than an hour, you only need to replenish fluids—water will do the trick without the added calories.

Q: We usually have soda, sports drinks, and fruit juice in the fridge. Which is healthiest?

A: In a word: None. Soda, juice, and sports drinks usually have tons of calories but little nutritional value. Instead of these, try stocking your fridge with fruit-flavored seltzers or water. If you don't like the taste of water, add lemon (or a cucumber slice in a pinch). Or try packets of sugar-free iced tea or lemonade that you mix with a glass of water.

a healthy diet

Q: Is flavored vitamin water as healthy or healthier than plain water?

A Drinking flavored water is better than drinking *no* water, but plain water is best because it's calorie-free (a 20-ounce bottle of of vitamin water can have more calories than a can of soda!) Don't like plain water? Pick a flavored one with fewer than 10 calories per serving.

Q: Is bottled water safer or better for you than tap water?

A The Environmental Protection Agency sets safety standards for tap water, and the Food and Drug Administration regulates bottled water—so both are safe to drink. Both types of water are allowed to have *trace* amounts of contaminants, so neither is safer than the other. All bottled water is not the same though. Purified water (like Dasani) is basically filtered tap water. Spring water (like Poland Spring) and artesian water (like Fiji) come from sources inside the earth. Mineral water (like Evian) is also from a source in the earth, but it has more natural minerals than spring water. They may taste different, but they're all safe, so choose the water that tastes best to you. If you'd rather not spend money, tap is of course, on tap!

portion control

Q My friend and I have a disagreement about how much pasta you're supposed to eat at a meal. She thinks it's only a scoop, but if that's true, why do I always get so much more when I eat out?

A We hate to disappoint you, but your friend is right. One scoop (about ½ cup) may seem like a small amount, but it's actually what the USDA considers a serving of grain, rice, or pasta. Unfortunately, the average amount of pasta that American restaurants serve is almost *four* times that much! Here's a way to make pasta a healthier restaurant choice: Divide the portion in half when it's served and ask the server to wrap up one half for you to bring home.

a healthy diet

Q: For snacking, what's better to do—buy small snack-size bags, or measure out your own portion from a larger bag?

A: Eating from larger bags or containers makes you more likely to consume too many calories. But it's cheaper to buy larger bags, so if you want to save money—and calories!—prevent overeating by dividing snacks into single-serving baggies. Snacks should be about 15 chips or 2 regular-sized cookies (100–200 calories). Better yet, scrap the salty, greasy snacks altogether and munch on grapes or baby carrots instead!

Q: I like to eat big portions. If I don't fill my plate, I don't feel full, and then I end up snacking between meals. At this rate, I'm afraid I'll never lose weight. What should I do?

A: You'd rather eat a big portion of anything rather than a tiny portion of a food you love. That's okay when you're eating things like vegetables, but not when it comes to junk food. If you need to eat big, bulk up your meals with veggies. If you're having macaroni and cheese for dinner, mix in a cup of steamed broccoli. Your portion will become larger and everything still tastes cheesy—but it's much healthier this way! Also, go for sides that come as single servings, like corn on the cob, a baked potato, or a yam, instead of pasta or mashed potatoes. This will help you control the amount you consume.

CG! TIP: Always serve yourself small portions. If you're still hungry 20 minutes after you eat, you can always go back for seconds.

Q: How do I know how much of something I'm supposed to eat?

A. Read food labels. The serving size listed right at the top is the recommended amount to eat of any food, and the amount the manufacturer is basing all the other nutritional information on. If the serving size is 10 chips, and you scarf down 30, you have to multiply the other percentages on the label by three.

a healthy diet

healthy habits

Q: My family and I eat most of our meals in front of the TV, but I can't help but feel this isn't very healthy for us. Am I right?

A: Probably. Some studies show that you eat mindlessly while watching TV, so you're more likely to overeat when you dine in front of the tube. Maybe it's time you made a big change in your family's routine. Try to institute a no-TV rule during dinner with your parents, and then use the time to learn more about one another. (Try asking conversation-starting questions like, "If you could travel anywhere, where would you go?") Not only will you end up skinnier, but you'll be more closely connected to family members!

CG! TIP: In the mood for candy? Pick the one that lasts longest—a minute spent with one sucking candy on your tongue is better than a minute popping a bagful of Skittles nonstop!

Q **I want to eat less at meals, but my mother feels like she has to serve everyone's food and then she expects me to clean my plate—even if I'm not that hungry. What can I do?**

A You're totally right about wanting to be in control of what you eat, and that you probably do eat more now than you would if you served yourself. And if you're required to clean your plate, even if you're not hungry, that's a surefire way to get saddled with saddlebags. Your mom's not trying to fatten you up. Remember, your parents work hard for the money to buy groceries, and they also work hard to prepare meals and put them on the table. They don't want to see their efforts wasted, and who can blame them? But that doesn't mean you need to bloat up to make them happy. Just politely explain to your mom that you're trying to eat less, and ask to serve yourself. Take small portions to start. If your family's worried about food going to waste because every bite doesn't get swallowed at that particular meal, suggest a leftovers night on Fridays, where you reheat the week's leftovers and serve them buffet style.

a healthy diet

Q **I eat so much faster than all my friends and I never feel full. And then I start picking off their plates. If I keep this up, I'm going to be a blimp by the time I graduate from high school. Help!**

A Eating fast is not good for you, but for more reasons than having the time to pick off your friends' plates. Try to slow yourself down. Why? Actually paying attention to what you're eating makes your food more filling. Think about it—you probably wouldn't finish off a tub of popcorn if you were sitting at a table doing nothing else, but you might eat that much during a movie without even realizing it. And since it takes 20 minutes for your brain to register what's in your stomach, eating slowly allows you to be a better judge of how much food it takes for you to feel full.

snack attack

Q: I know my favorite after-school snack isn't healthy, but I can't help myself!

A: If you crave foods that aren't good for you, and indulge all the time, you know what's going to happen. Junk food is fine, but only once in a while! Try to eat healthfully during the week and indulge those must-haves on weekends only. Whatever you do, don't stop eating your faves altogether—that'll just make you crave them even more. Balance your diet by eating less of the food group that includes your favorite foods throughout the day. For example, if you must have a bagel for breakfast, eat fewer starchy foods at lunch (try vegetable soup instead of pizza).

a healthy diet

Q **I get so hungry before dinner, I just have to eat a snack. What can I easily make that's healthy too?**

A Instead of potato or tortilla chips, make your own savory snack with our homemade Pita Chips and Fruit Salsa (see page 22 for the easy recipe). Need to grab a snack while you're running out the door? A handful of almonds will curb that after-school hunger. In addition to being full of flavor, they have the perfect combination of carbs, protein, and monosaturated fat, which can boost your concentration and help you study—not to mention plenty of zinc, which helps your brain gather and process information. You can also try natural peanut butter (it has a lot less sugar and salt than regular supermarket brands) slathered on a whole-wheat mini bagel or cut up a Granny Smith apple and dip it into a cup of nonfat yogurt. If you're looking for a treat to satisfy your sweet tooth, try yogurt and fruit combos instead of chocolate ice cream. Our Fake Banana Cream Pie is a good source of calcium and protein—in fact, it's a snack so balanced, it's like a mini-meal. Here's how to make it: Peel one banana and cut it into slices. Break two graham crackers into four smaller crackers each. Place a few banana slices on each cracker and open a 4-ounce container of low-fat vanilla yogurt. Then add 2 tablespoons yogurt to each of your "pies" and garnish with a sprinkle of cinnamon. See page 34 for another fruit-and-yogurt treat recipe: our delicious Strawberry-Yogurt Parfait. Yum!

CG! TIP: During the day, snack on brightly colored fruits and vegetables—like berries, carrot sticks, or apples—to add antioxidants to your diet.

a healthy diet

diet myths

Q **I need to go on a diet, but I'm just not ready to give up eating everything I love. What can I do?**

A Keeping your body healthy doesn't mean you have to give up your favorite food altogether or count every calorie. Life without chocolate? What's the point? In fact, depriving yourself of your favorite foods will only make you crave them more. If you're in the mood for chocolate, have something small. Savoring a few small chocolate candies can satisfy a chocolate craving (and keep you from scarfing down five chocolate chip cookies later).

Q **My friends have all decided to skip eating lunch to keep their weight down. I know you have to eat breakfast to get yourself going in the morning, and dinner you usually have to eat with your parents, so I guess if you're looking to cut calories, skipping lunch really is the only solution. Right?**

A *Wrong.* Skipping meals is the worst thing you can do when you're trying to lose weight. When you skip meals, any meals, your body automatically responds as if it's starving. Even if you know you'll eat again, your body fears you may not and slows your metabolism to conserve calories. The next time you eat, you're likely to store those calories as fat, since your body is saving up for going without food again.

a healthy diet

Q: I always eat diet foods but can't seem to ever lose weight. Why not?

A: Eating healthfully can be tricky. Remember: Just because an item is labeled "low fat" or "low carb" doesn't mean it's the best choice. It might have more sugar or salt to make up for the ingredients that were removed. Fat-free snacks and some diet nutrition bars often contain more sugar (and sometimes more calories!) than the regular versions. Plus, foods with a little fat take longer to digest than fat-free foods, so they taste better and keep you full longer.

Q: There are so many different diet plans, I have no idea what I should be cutting out and what I should be bulking up on. Help!

A: With all the different diets out there, it can be tough to figure out what's truly good for you. But the key to eating healthy is not cutting stuff out—it's eating just enough vitamin-rich whole foods, like veggies, lean meat, and multigrain bread, and cutting back on foods that have been processed, like frozen meals and packaged snacks. And if you like to indulge occasionally when you eat out, go for it! Just keep your diet balanced by eating better when you have meals at home.

key ingredients

Q I try to read food labels on products before I buy or eat them, but I don't know what a lot of the information on them means. Can you give me a rundown?

A Sure. You probably already know that the serving size is the recommended amount to eat, and the servings per package means how many times you should be diving back into the bag to finish it. Now here's some stuff you may not know: The Calories and Calories From Fat sections show you how much energy your body gets from a serving of this food, and how much comes from fat. On average, you should be eating about 2,200 calories per day, and 30 percent (or 73 grams) of them should be coming from fat. At least 55–60 percent should be coming from complex carbs (about 302–330). Percent (%) of Daily Values shows what percentage of the total recommended daily intake of each nutrient you're getting in a serving of this food. In general, 5 percent is low and 20 percent is high. So balance what you eat each day and try not to exceed 100 percent of anything. The Total values are the same on every label. They show the amount of fat, cholesterol, sodium, fiber, and carbs you should eat per day, based on a 2,000- or 2,500-calorie-a-day diet. If your total calorie count is somewhere in between, just estimate up or down.

a healthy diet

CG! TIP: Eat light-meat tuna or salmon three times a week. These cold-water fish have omega-3 fatty acids, which boost brain power!

Q I've heard a lot about minerals, but I'm not exactly sure what they are and how the body uses them. Can you explain—and also tell me how I can get what I need into my diet?

A Minerals help with everything from paying attention in class to easing cramps. (Who knew?) Here's how to get enough of the three you really need! You need about 15mg per day of iron, which helps your red blood cells carry oxygen to your muscles and organs, and keeps you more alert so you can pay attention in class. A big source of iron is lean beef (about 3mg per serving), but fortified cereals, beans, spinach, eggs, and blackberries are also good sources. Zinc helps you grow and mature physically (it helps you get your period and develop breasts) and also keeps your immune system strong. The 9mgs you need a day can come from lots of sources, including lean meats, nuts, and fortified cereals. If you're a vegetarian, take note: You need up to 13mgs of zinc a day, as the body doesn't absorb plant sources of zinc as well as it does animal sources. See pages 58-59 for mineral-rich alternatives. Calcium is one of the most important minerals and you should get it any way you can! It's crucial to bone formation, which continues till you're 18. It also keeps your teeth strong and has been shown to ease PMS cramps. The whopping 1,300mg you need per day can come from milk and fortified juices (about 300mg per cup!) as well as from other dairy, fortified cereals, spinach, and broccoli.

Q: I sometimes get obsessed with certain foods and eat only those. Is that bad for me?

A. Possibly, but it really depends on what you're eating. Since you tend to eat the same stuff all the time, you probably get lots of some vitamins but not enough of others. So alternate your usual meals with ones that contain foods from different groups. If you always have dairy and grains for lunch (like grilled cheese), try a lunch that has protein and veggies (like a grilled chicken salad). You probably eat more grains than produce, so try a new fruit or veggie each week. Who knows? You may like kiwi slices as much as candy!

a healthy diet

Q: My stomach always feels puffy, even after I exercise. Why?

A Chances are that it isn't fat you're feeling, but bloating or gas, caused by eating high-fiber foods, swallowing air (by chewing gum or eating too fast), or retaining fluids. Try these tips for two weeks and you'll start to get flatter! Replace carbonated drinks with water or veggie juice. Instead of chewing gum, try mouthwash or a mint. Replace dried fruit with fresh—like berries or melon. Avoid refried beans and opt for grilled chicken or tofu. Lastly, don't flavor your food with salt; fresh herbs like basil or unsalted spices will prevent you from retaining water.

Q: I've heard that apples can help ease gastric problems. Is that true?

A: The expression "An apple a day keeps the doctor away" isn't really that far from the truth, especially when it comes to keeping your digestive system running smoothly. A single large apple has 5 grams of fiber—about 25 percent of what doctors recommend that you eat each day. It's this fiber that helps move food through your digestive tract more quickly while preventing constipation (because it makes you go to the bathroom more regularly). But stomach-smart as apples may be, if you find yourself suffering from any kind of digestive problem—like heartburn, constipation, bloating, or gas—check in with your doctor. She may prescribe a medication or help you trace the problem to a specific food intolerance. In many situations, simply cutting certain foods out of your diet may ease gastric problems.

a healthy diet

veg fact & fiction

Q I've been thinking about becoming a vegetarian, but my mom's worried that I may be losing out on some important vitamins if I cut meat and fish out of my diet. How can I eat the way I want but still make my mom happy?

A The first thing you should do before giving up meat is consult a registered dietitian. In fact, that's a good practice any time you're thinking of a drastic change in diet. Now, you're probably going to hate hearing this, but your mom is absolutely right to be worried about you getting proper nutrition. You're still growing after all. If you really want to become a healthy herbivore, you need to make sure that you're getting certain vital nutrients that you used to rely on meat and fish for.

- One of the biggest ones you'll be missing is protein. Muscles, organs, antibodies (infection fighters), and hemoglobin (which oxygenates the body) are made of protein. To make sure you get this in your diet, eat lots of brown rice, beans, soy, eggs, dairy, and nuts.
- During your period, you lose lots of iron. If you don't replace it, you may become anemic, which will make you feel really tired.

To get iron in your diet without consuming meat, eat plenty of fortified grains and cereals, dark leafy greens, beans, and peas.

- Calcium, crucial to building bone mass, is deposited into your bone bank through your early 30s. That means you want to get as much of this nutrient as possible now! Maximize calcium intake by eating lots of dark leafy greens, dairy, and calcium-fortified foods (check labels).
- Zinc works hand-in-hand with iron; your body uses it to heal wounds and repair muscles and tissue. (It's also great for clearing your skin.) Good sources of zinc include peas, beans, brown rice, spinach, nuts, tofu, and tempeh. Vitamin B_{12} is good for red blood cells and your nervous system. Get this essential nutrient from fortified foods, eggs, and dairy products.

Here's another tip for a boost of nutrients: Use a cast-iron skillet when cooking, so more iron will get into your food. Also, when you do make the change, be sure to eliminate meat gradually. Adopt your new diet for just a few days at first, and work from there. Drop red meat first, then pork and poultry, then finally, fish. Visit vrg.org for recipes and more information.

CG! TIP: Look for iron-packed lentil and chickpea recipes at vegweb.com

a healthy diet

Q: I want to become a vegetarian because I think it will be a great way for me to lose weight. What do you think?

A: Losing weight is not a great reason to become a vegetarian. These diets don't mean weight loss—in fact, you could gain weight if you sub high-cal foods like fries for meat. Becoming a vegetarian is actually a serious life choice that will mean making changes that aren't as simple as just skipping meat. Vegetarians have to eat a wide variety of foods to get the nutrients they need. That can be difficult if you're a picky eater! Also, if you don't like to plan, it's not going to be that easy for you. Being a veg means thinking ahead so you can eat right each day and be sure there are options when you eat out. Vegetarianism can be healthy, but it's not the next quick diet fix!

Q: What's the difference between the types of vegetarians? I've heard that if I am a certain type of vegetarian, I can eat fish. Is that true?

A: Actually, there are four types of vegetarians—and not one of them eats fish. Which of these you decide to become depends on why you're adopting the vegetarian diet:

- *Lacto-ovo vegetarians* eat only plant foods, plus eggs and dairy (milk, cheese, butter, and yogurt). Because it's the least restrictive of all the vegetarian diets, the only nutrient you'll have to worry about not getting enough of is iron.
- *Lacto vegetarians* eat only plant foods and dairy—no eggs. If you're on this diet, be sure to have at least two to three servings of protein a day, as well as iron-rich foods.
- *Ovo vegetarians* eat only plant foods and eggs—no dairy, so the primary nutritional concerns with this eating style are iron, calcium, and vitamin D.
- *Vegans* eat strictly plant foods, so many essential nutrients are missing from this diet. Be sure to take supplements to get those necessary nutrients.

a healthy diet

Q: What can I eat to make up for the protein and calcium that may be missing in my diet as a vegetarian?

A Our Easy Vegetarian Stuffed Pita has almost half the protein you need in a day, plus it's got whole grains and veggies. Follow package directions for microwaving 1 frozen Gardenburger. Once it's heated, cut it into bite-size pieces. Slice open 1 whole-wheat pita pocket and spread 1 tablespoon prepared hummus inside. Stuff in the burger pieces, 1 tablespoon shredded cheese (any kind), and your favorite sandwich vegetables (lettuce, tomato, onions, etc.). Then dig in! For calcium, try our Chocolate Strawberry Smoothie. Cut 6 strawberries into small pieces and place in blender. Add 4 ice cubes, ½ cup skim milk, ½ cup low-fat chocolate frozen yogurt, and 1 packet Carnation Instant Breakfast. Blend and drink!

Q **I'm a vegetarian, so I typically eat rice, pasta, or potatoes for dinner. How can I make my diet more well-rounded—without adding too many extra calories?**

A While all these foods are healthy (especially when you choose brown rice and whole-grain pasta), they all belong to the same food group: grains. To make sure you're getting *all* the nutrients you need, you must eat foods from at least three food groups at every meal (think grains, vegetables, and beans or other protein). Try pasta with lentil (protein) tomato sauce, or a stir-fry with brown rice, veggies, and tofu (protein).

a healthy diet

Q: My family eats meat, but I don't. I just eat the side dishes, but these don't seem as satisfying. Any suggestions?

A: Going veggie doesn't mean you're just not eating meat; it means you replace meat with other protein-rich foods—and we don't mean powders or pills when we say "foods." Keep veggie or soy burgers in the freezer so you can heat them up quickly and have them with the side dishes, print out recipes from vrg.org or vegweb.com and offer to make them for your whole family, or whip up a veg entrée (like eggplant parmigiana) on the weekend and heat it up for weekday meals.

Q: I take vitamins and protein supplements because I don't eat meat. Isn't that enough?

A: While it's great that you realize a diet without meat may be low in protein and iron, vitamins and supplements are not a quick fix for a poor diet. Plus, eating a variety of vegetarian foods is a better way to get protein and vitamins because it ensures you're getting all the other nutrients you need as well. Peanut butter, beans, soy milk, and fortified cereals are good sources of iron and protein.

a healthy diet

healthy meals on the go

Q **My schedule is so packed, I barely have time to breathe during the day—let alone stop for lunch. I already know skipping meals is not a healthy way to go, so what should I eat for lunch that I can make quickly and will fill me up till dinner?**

A Try a tuna salad whole-wheat pita. Before you leave for school in the morning, toss together the tuna salad. Take a 4-ounce can of tuna (if you don't like tuna, substitute with diced, grilled chicken breast) and mix it with ¼ cup plain, low-fat yogurt, 2 tablespoons diced red onion, 2 tablespoons diced celery, 2 tablespoons diced carrots, 1 teaspoon lime juice, and salt and pepper to taste. Put this in one container. Next, cut a whole-wheat pita in half, and put this in another container. In a separate container, place 6 leaves of washed Bibb lettuce. When you're ready to eat, throw the sandwich together by adding lettuce and tuna salad to each pita half—and voilà! Bon appetit!

CG! TIP: Strawberries are a great source of vitamin C and fiber!

Q: I'm looking for a quick, healthy lunch I can have on weekends. Any ideas?

A: Try this chicken wrap—it will give you nearly two servings of veggies (you need to eat five servings a day), while the lemon juice, herbs, and spices add flavor without fat. Blend together ⅛ teaspoon each of basil, oregano, garlic powder, and black pepper, then sprinkle them on both sides of a 3-ounce chicken breast. Spray a nonstick skillet with cooking spray, heat about 2 minutes over medium-high heat, then add chicken. Reduce heat to medium and cook chicken about 14 minutes, turning it to brown both sides. Remove from heat, cut the center to make sure it's cooked (it should be opaque, not pink), and slice it into thin strips. Place chicken on a 6-inch whole-grain tortilla, top with ⅔ cup shredded romaine lettuce, ¼ cup shredded carrot, and ¼ cup cucumber, peeled and thinly sliced. Drizzle with 1 teaspoon fresh lemon juice and ½ teaspoon olive oil. Then fold up the sides and enjoy!

a healthy diet

Q: I have an after-school job and I usually don't get home until 9 or 9:30, which is really late to eat. What should I eat for dinner?

A: Here's one of our favorites. It's quick, easy, healthy, and did we mention yummy? You'll need: 1 teaspoon olive oil, a 4-ounce boneless breast of chicken, ½ cup of fruit or regular salsa, a handful of mixed greens, ½ cup uncooked brown rice, and 1 cup low-fat ice cream. Preheat oven to 400 degrees. Preheat oven-safe skillet on stove and add oil. Brown the chicken over medium heat for 1½ minutes on each side, then place chicken (still in skillet) in the oven. Bake 15 to 20 minutes, until it's completely cooked. (Cut through the breast to see if it's done. Still pink? Keep cooking until it's white.) While chicken cooks, make a side of brown rice following the directions on the box. Slice chicken breast into 5 or 6 pieces and place on top of greens. Top with salsa and enjoy. Then feed your sweet tooth with low-fat ice cream for dessert!

CG! TIP: Find quick, lean beef recipes at beefitswhatsfordinner.com.

weight-loss dilemmas

Q: I've heard that there's a connection between not sleeping and gaining weight. Is that true?

A: Recent research is beginning to prove more and more that when you don't get enough sleep, you put yourself at risk for becoming obese. Why? Blame it on hormones. When you sleep, levels of the hormone leptin, which signals when the body needs or does not need more food, rise. When you don't get enough sleep, or sleep is interrupted, leptin levels are low, and your body thinks it needs more calories. You'll feel hungry, and therefore eat more. The key? Get more sleep. If you can't get the recommended nine solid hours, try squeezing in a nap here and there. Remember—sleep deprivation does more than make you chubby—it also results in poor concentration, crankiness, and a weakened immune system.

> **CG! TIP: Multivitamins and supplements are not a substitute for the vitamins and minerals you get from food. So eat up!**

a healthy diet

Q **I'm trying to lose weight in a healthy way, but even though I just eat what's on my plate, never go back for seconds, and don't snack between meals, it's still not working. Why not?**

A Even without knowing it, you could still be overeating. Really! Did you know that most restaurants serve 30 to 50 percent more food than you need so that you feel like you're getting your money's worth? And even at home, you may be eating 25 percent too much because restaurants have distorted your view of proper portion sizes. What are the right amounts of food? For lean chicken, meat or fish, about 3 ounces—or the size of a cosmetic compact. Baked potato or cooked rice? About ½ cup—or the size of a tennis ball. For cheese, about 1 ounce, or a 1-inch cosmetic wedge. For salad dressing, about 1 tablespoon—about as much as a bottle of nail polish. Once you learn what a healthy portion looks like, you can eat the amounts you need to be healthy and feel great.

Q **I'm always on a diet, but I can't seem to lose any weight. I eat every good thing there is, but still the pounds stay on, not off. What can I do?**

A Sounds like you're eating healthily, but you need to also make sure you're controlling your portions. If you are, you may not be doing enough physical activity to balance out how much you're eating. Balancing good eating habits with working out is the best way to maintain your healthy weight. Learn more about this in Chapter 2, Work It Out.

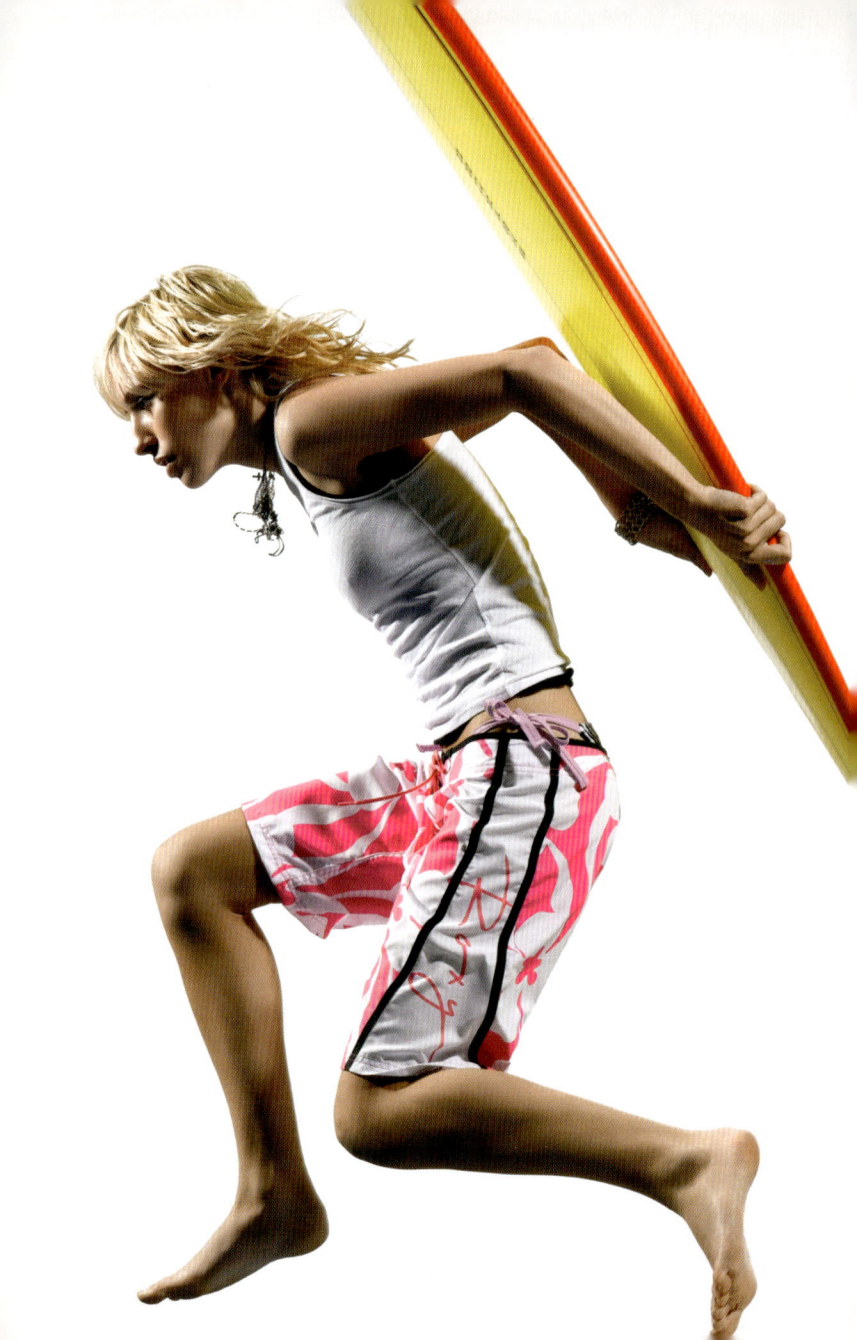

chapter 2

work it out

What you eat is only part of the equation when you want to be fit. In fact, regular exercise is the only way to maintain a healthy weight. In addition to burning excess calories and strengthening your body, exercise also makes you feel good. So get up off that couch, CosmoGIRL!, and check out what we've been telling your fellow CG!s about how to work that body!

work it out

fab abs

Q: My stomach always looks so fat. What can I do to make it flatter?

A: A lot of the time, your stomach will look fat—not because it actually is, but because of the way you're holding your body. Don't believe us? Stand sideways in front of a mirror. Now, straighten your body, pulling back your shoulders and holding your abs firm and tight. See the difference? What you want to focus on is not necessarily flattening your tummy, but strengthening your core muscles so you're always "pulling it in." Sit-ups and leg circles are just some of the ways to work your body to the core.

Q: I do so many crunches a day, but how can I know I'm doing them the right way so I'm not wasting my time?

A: While you're doing crunches, or any exercises for that matter, keep your abs pulled in tight and contracted. To get an idea of what it feels like, stand up, place your palms on your stomach, and cough. Feel that tightening? That's what your abs should feel like when you engage them in exercises. Also, for each set you do, do as many reps as you can while maintaining the correct form. We suggest 10-15 reps, but your number may be different for each move.

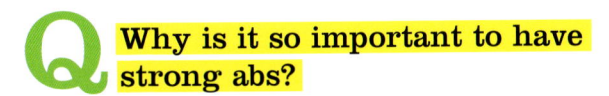

Q: Why is it so important to have strong abs?

A: The muscles that make up your core—your abs, obliques, and lower back muscles—provide power for all your movements. When you strengthen your core, your posture improves and all your other muscles work more efficiently, which helps prevent injuries from sports and other exercises. Bonus: Having a strong core is the first step to getting the oh-so-sexy six-pack you've been working toward!

work it out

no butts about it!

Q: I have a really big butt. How can I tone it down so it looks more like Beyoncé's?

A: Try lunges, squats, and kicks to give yourself the best booty. Don't forget that you can turn it into a calorie-burning cardio workout by jumping rope for five minutes before you begin, then doing 100 skips of a jump rope between moves.

fitting in fitness

Q **I have so much going on right now, I can't even think about working out. But I know I need to exercise somehow. What can you recommend?**

A We know you're busy, but keep this in mind: The one thing that's been proven to help you deal with all that stress is exercise! Not only does it make your body look good, it makes you feel good by increasing your energy level, reducing tension, and even making you happier in general. So make exercise part of your life now!

work it out

Q: I'd like to get into a fitness routine, but especially in the summer, I just get so lazy! What can I do to jump-start an exercise plan?

A: Even if you let most of the summer go by without moving a muscle, starting a physical activity now will get you motivated for later. It's a positive cycle that works like this: You start exercising (like jumping rope or taking brisk walks), and your brain releases feel-good, stress-fighting endorphins to your nervous system. This means that while you're working out you can more easily focus. In short, happy body means happy mind.

Q **I have a hard time staying motivated once I start working out. I'll be excited about it for the first week or so, but then too many other things get in the way. Any suggestions on how to stick with a routine?**

A Consider keeping a workout log or chart. You can use it to write down your goals and see what you've achieved each time you exercise. It's amazing how much motivation you'll get just from writing something down! Also, try to exercise at the same time every day. That way, you can make it part of your routine, like taking a shower or brushing your teeth. It will become more of a habit and less of a chore in no time!

work it out

Q: I usually only have time to exercise at night, around bedtime. Is that all right?

A: Absolutely—*when* you work out has no effect on how many calories you burn or how toned your muscles become. The important thing is how regularly you work out: For best results, doctors say you should aim for at least 30 minutes of heart-pumping cardio activity every day. That said, we've got two warnings about evening sweat sessions: (1) Stay safe! Use an exercise video at home or go to your local gym. If you must run outside, run with at least one buddy. (2) Late-night workouts may make you feel too revved up to sleep. If this happens, cool off during the last 10 minutes of your session with some gentle stretches or yoga moves. Ahhhhh! Sweet dreams, fit girl!

Q I really want to start working out more, but I don't have the money to join a gym and I get so bored with all those machines anyway. Any ideas?

A Why confine yourself to a gym when you can work off calories in Nature's own gym? If you don't live near hiking trails, go for a brisk walk through a safe park path or a hilly section of your neighborhood. The best part about it—membership is free!

CG! TIP: Meet a friend at the mall and power-walk the length of the mall twice before you shop.

work it out

run with it!

Q: I want to get into running, but I'm not sure how to go about it. Do you have any good tips for setting up a running program, sticking with it, and not hurting myself while I'm at it?

A: When you're just beginning to run, don't push yourself too hard. The key is to prepare your body for running, and not to overdo it, which can cause you to burn out or even hurt yourself. Even when you've been at it a while, run only 3 times a week (no more than 4) for 30 minutes, including warm-up. Your muscles need rest to relax and get stronger, so take a day off between each run. You'll become a better runner that way and want to stick with it. Stay motivated by running with a friend. You can keep each other entertained—and as you get better and better, you can start testing your competitive sides! Now, if you're running alone, you're going to get bored easily if all you're thinking about is the end of the run. Instead, focus on how your body moves and take in the scenery. You'll have more fun! Don't get too discouraged by thinking you should be able to run faster or farther. Always warm up by walking fast at least 5 minutes before you run. When you're first starting out, try intervals. Run for 3-5 minutes, then walk fast for 1-2, and repeat until you hit

30 minutes. If you're breathing hard, or if something hurts, slow down. Do only what feels right—that's how you become a runner for life. Eat foods rich in iron (chicken, soy products, dark leafy greens), potassium (potatoes, bananas, apples), and vitamin B_{12} (fortified cereals, meats, milk) to give you the fuel you need for endurance. Finally, know your body. If you feel faint while running, you're probably dehydrated. Be sure to drink water throughout the day to keep hydrated. If you're fatigued after running for less than 15 minutes, add more iron and vitamin B_{12} to your diet.

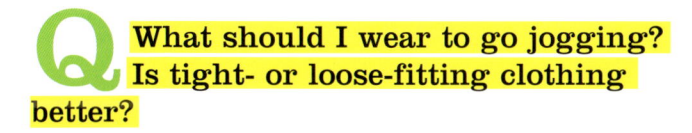

Q: What should I wear to go jogging? Is tight- or loose-fitting clothing better?

A When you run, wear stretchy, fitted—but not tight—shirts, and shorts or pants that won't get in the way of body movement. Also, get a sports bra labeled "Dri-Fit"—it'll really absorb your sweat. Do jumping jacks in the dressing room to make sure the bra supports but isn't so tight under your arms or around your torso that it's uncomfortable.

work it out

Q: Does it really matter what kind of sneakers I wear when I go jogging?

A Absolutely. Think about how much impact you're putting on your legs—your knees and ankles and feet. Shop for running sneakers at a specialty running store, where experts can help you avoid injury by telling you whether your arch is high or low, how flexible your feet are, and whether your feet roll inward or outward. Tell the salesperson that you're a beginning runner—she'll ask you to walk around the store to see how your feet land. She'll pick out a few pairs for you to try on so you can see what's right for you. Sneakers designed for stability give support and cushioning, and are great starter shoes for beginners who aren't sure how their feet move. Cushion sneakers are less supportive than ones tailored to stability, but because they're soft, they're good for street runners or people with strong feet. Motion-control sneakers support the side of your feet, keeping them from rolling too far inward or outward (if that's a problem for you).

> **CG! TIP:** Before working out, always warm up by jogging or jumping rope for five minutes.

cool cardio

Q: I hate exercising. I always have and always will. I never play sports, and I sometimes lie to the school nurse about having bad period cramps so I can sit out gym class. I know I should be doing something, but what?

A: Here are some cool ways you can exercise and not even notice you're doing it. Try Bikram yoga. Practiced in up to 105-degree heat, it helps you achieve physical and emotional balance. Or take a hike. Find cool paths to explore in your area. Take a trapeze class and learn to fly like an acrobat. Pedal with a partner. The same old bike paths look different on a bicycle built for two, so rent a tandem bike and pick up a friend (one with stamina!). Whack some balls. Head to a golf driving range and take lessons. You'll relieve stress, plus you'll pick up a skill that will impress everyone. Load black-and-white film into your camera and take photos of your neighborhood. You'll get some funky shots—and the more scouting of locations you do, the more walking—exercise—you'll get in!

CG! TIP: Jumping outdoors on a hard surface? Soften your landing (and save your knees) by putting down a gym mat.

work it out

Q I know cardio's important, but I can never get motivated to go to the gym and exercise bikes and treadmills are so boring. Jogging seems so time-consuming, and I'm not really interested in any sports. Is there any other way I can get my cardio in, without having to move around too much?

A Here are some of our favorite ways to exercise without working up a sweat. First, hide the remote so you actually have to get up off the couch to change channels. It turns channel surfing into exercise. When you pull into a parking lot, choose a spot as far from your destination as possible. (Just make sure it's a well-lit spot.) Not only will you get exercise as you make your way to the entrance, you can make a quick exit when you're through. And finally, any time you talk on your cell phone, walk around—even if it's just walking around your room. To see how much cardio that adds to your day, just check out the daily airtime on your phone bill!

Q: I've heard dancing can be great exercise. I hate most kinds of exercise, but I really love dancing. Can you give me any tips for making dance my workout?

A: Dancing is an excellent way to get your heart pumping and burn calories while toning your arms, legs, and abs. Dance moves may seem hard at first, but once they click you'll know them for life! Soon you'll have the energy of a dancer, plus a rockin' toned body! Choreographed workouts can be so much fun you won't realize they're also killer cardio sessions. You can sign up for dance classes, but if you're short on time and money, pay close attention to the routines in your favorite music videos and try to memorize them. Incorporate these into your workout, and you'll start seeing results in no time—and you'll be having a great time while you're at it!

work it out

Q **I want to be able to wear a bathing suit without scaring everyone off the beach. Are there any special tips you can give me for toning those parts that show when I'm in a bikini?**

A The best answer for getting bikini fit is to do a routine that works on all parts of your body, not just your abs or legs. Sure, your belly, which isn't usually exposed, will be on full display, but there are other parts of you that are going to show, and by working these out and toning them up, you'll attract more attention to them and all the focus won't go on the parts of you that aren't as easy to firm. Take your arms, for instance. Toned biceps are sexy and can steal the show—take a look at Jennifer Garner's or Jessica Biel's arms! They're also easy to get. Regular bicep curls will give you nice definition—not to mention strength.

Q **The cheerleaders in my school all look really fit, and I was wondering if it was because they're all on crazy diets, or if cheerleading really is better exercise than I ever thought it was.**

A Make no mistake about it: Cheerleaders work it—and hard! Anyone who says cheerleading isn't a sport hasn't been to a conditioning session. Think about it. Cheerleaders have to be amazingly fit to do everything from flipping to hoisting each other up in the air. Their moves can give you a rockin' body—after all, who can pull off a short skirt better than a cheerleader?

work it out

Q: I've heard that listening to music while you exercise makes your workout more effective. Is this true?

A: Actually, yes. Listening to music when you exercise will not only motivate you to action, it will actually make you exercise harder—even if you're just taking a walk. Not only are the beats strong and driving, but the music can help you block out distractions and really get into the zone. Music is so effective for exercising, in fact, that there are whole workouts designed around music, like punk rock aerobics, designed by instructors to save themselves—and you—from all of the lame, boring workouts out there. Who says punk's just for moshing? Crank up the music and do some heart-pumping, muscle-toning moves for a great body!

CG! TIP: After a workout, be sure to give yourself a five-minute cooldown period to give your heart rate a chance to return to normal.

Q: I want to start exercising at home, but don't want to spend a fortune on weights. What can I substitute?

A: There are lots of things you can safely use as weights. For 3–5 pound hand weights use two 1-liter bottles filled with water.

Q: I get so stressed out before finals. I've heard that exercise can help me relax—is that true?

A: Exercise is a great stress reliever and mood elevator—and kickboxing is one of the best stress busters we know. Do you ever get so stressed out that you just want to hit something? Here's your chance! Kickboxing is great for toning your arms, abs, butt and legs—and you can't beat it for delivering a knock-out blow to all that tension you've been carrying around. In addition to being a great cardio workout, it builds balance, strength, and endurance. Do a 25-minute workout three times a week and you'll look and feel stronger in about four weeks.

work it out

aches and pains

Q: Whenever I run, I get really bad side cramps. Is there anything I can do to prevent them—or make them go away?

A: The cramps are probably caused by one (or more) of the following: dehydration (not drinking enough water during the day), irregular breathing (people often forget to breathe during workouts), or overexertion (simply pushing yourself too hard). To reduce cramping, drink two glasses of water about 30 minutes before you begin your workout, and train yourself to breathe rhythmically (turn down your MP3 player so you can hear your breath). To do this, walk briskly for 5 minutes, then ease into your stride, matching your breath to your running rhythm (for example, inhale when you step on your right foot and exhale when you step on it again). If you still feel a cramp coming on, you're pushing too hard. Walk until the cramp subsides, and slowly increase your pace when you're ready. Or try this method: Run for 10 minutes, power walk for another 10, and so on. It's a kinder way to train your body, and over time, you'll run longer, walk less—and forget all about those annoying cramps!

> **CG! TIP:** After cooling down, be sure to stretch your neck, arms, back, and legs.

Q **Every time I start a workout program, I end up hurting myself and then I have to stop for weeks—sometimes even months—at a time. How can I exercise without injury?**

A Stretching is key, and if you're hurting yourself all the time, you're probably forgetting to stretch—both before and after each workout. Hold each move for at least 30 seconds. For calves, step forward on your right foot with your knee bent. Your left leg should be behind you with your left heel planted. Learn forward slightly until you feel a stretch in your calf. Hold for 30 seconds, then switch sides. For your hamstrings, stretch your right leg in front of your body, with your foot flexed and your heel on the floor. Bend your left knee. Lean toward your left thigh until you feel a stretch in your right hamstring, then switch legs. To stretch those quads, bend your left knee and lift your foot behind you toward your butt. Hold it in place with your left hand. Bend your knees slightly and keep them in line with each other. Hold for 30 seconds, then switch legs. Always stretch your arms after using weights to prevent injury. Straighten your right arm. Hook your left elbow in front as you pull your right arm across your body. Hold for 10 seconds, then switch to stretch the other arm.

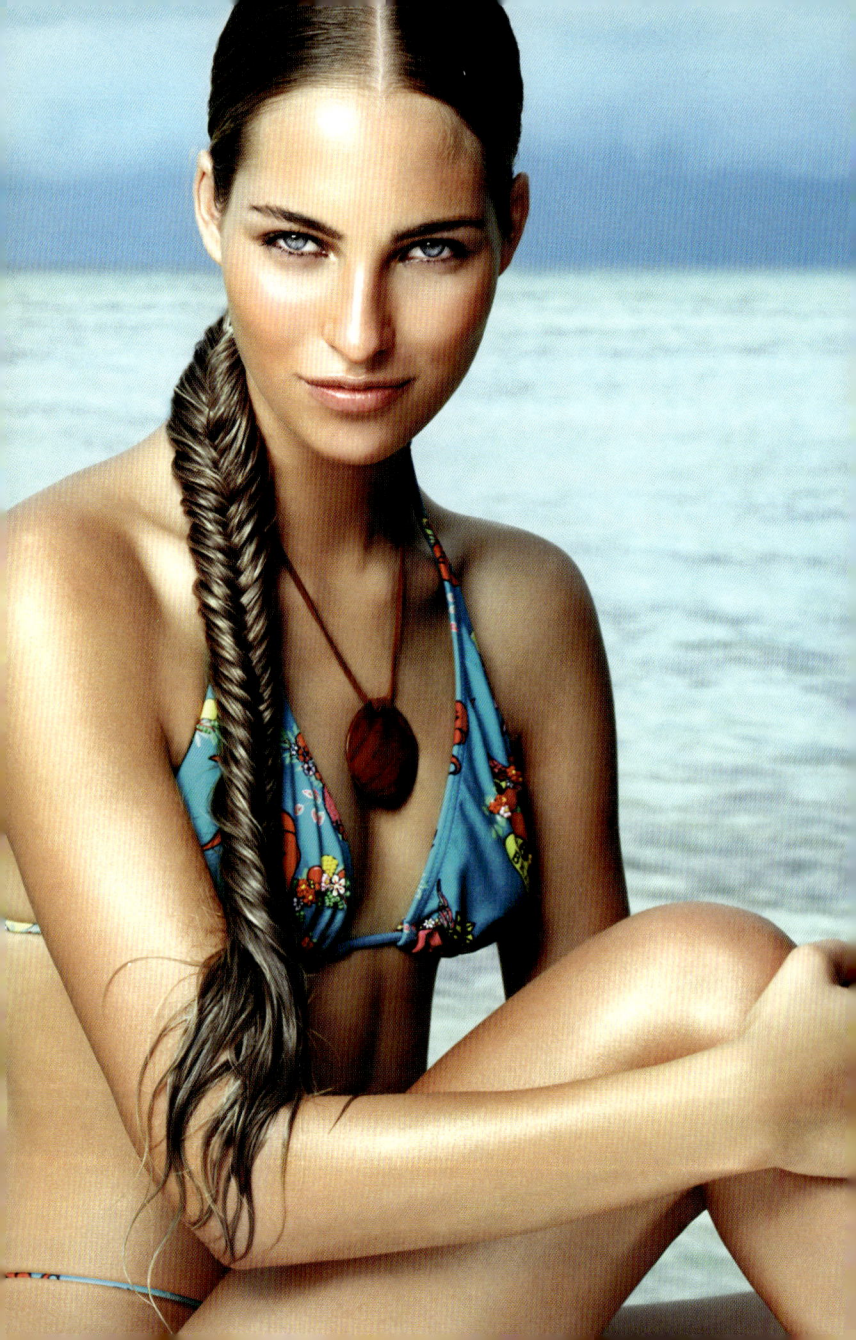

chapter 3

love your body

Guess what girls: Most of you are not as fat as you think you are! We get a lot of pressure in this society to be stick thin, but models and celebrities really are not the best measure. Sometimes it can feel like the pressure is coming from everywhere. Your fellow CG!s feel it too—so read on for our best love-your-body advice. And hey—want to know if you're the right weight? Make an appointment for a physical. Not only will your doctor know exactly how much you should weigh, but she can make healthy recommendations if you do need to gain or lose.

love your body

out of scale

Q **I have a little fat on my lower back—and huge thighs that never seem to get smaller. I want a body like a model. Any tips to help me get there?**

A Here's a start—models come in all shapes and sizes too. They just know how to emphasize their assets so you don't notice their less-than-perfect parts (and trust us—everybody has them). We know it's hard, but try not to be frustrated. If you are exercising regularly but aren't happy with the results, make some changes. Be sure your workout includes exercises that work your lower body, such as lunges, squats, and side kicks. And remember what we said about models—emphasize your assets. Choose a neckline that frames your pretty face; buy a new lipstick in the perfect shade of red; show off that beautiful smile. You'll be drawing people's attention to what you want them to see—you!

Q: I weigh myself every day and the number is never the same. I can't be more careful about watching my weight. What can I do to make sure the pounds stay off?

A: First and foremost: Don't weigh yourself. Ever. Your weight can change from day to day and hour to hour based on different factors (such as how hydrated you are), so obsessing over the number on the scale is pointless and can drive you insane! And because muscle weighs more than fat but takes up less space, the number on the scale can be misleading. A girl who wears a size 8 can actually weigh more than a girl who wears a size 12. Bottom line: Paying attention to how well your favorite clothes fit is a better way to keep track of how consistent your weight is.

love your body

clothes horse!

Q: I feel fat because my jeans look terrible on me—even though I know I'm wearing the right size. How can I fix this?

A: The trick is finding the cut and style that flatters you the most. Different styles from different brands will fit differently—even if they're the same size! So if you're full-figured, avoid tapered legs, which make hips and thighs appear larger than they are. Also, dark denim makes legs look sleeker. Many brands and stores have different jean lines designed for different figure types—some are even specially tailored to curvy women. These have more room in the hip and tush area, which makes them not only comfortable, but more flattering. Also: Avoid the dryer. Not only will it make jeans fade more quickly, but it causes them to shrink! Choose jeans with medium-sized back pockets placed on your butt or slightly above it. They draw the eye upward, giving your bum a visual lift.

Q: Why does it seem like clothes today are all tailored to fit small-chested, rail-thin girls? I have a little bulk on top, and these clothes look awful on me! Any advice?

A: First of all: You're not the problem here, okay? Sometimes clothes won't fit right on you because of the way they're cut. But don't worry, there are lots of options available. If you're bigger on top, try wearing scoop-neck shirts. They flatter your neckline and don't lay too tight across the chest. Avoid halter tops and crew necks; halter tops won't hold you correctly and a crew neck will actually make it look like you have more than you really do. Avoid knits that cling too tightly around the bust and, most importantly, invest in well-fitting bras.

Q: How can I draw attention away from my big booty?

A: Bring focus to the upper body with lace trim, embroidery, or other embellishment. An A-line skirt draws attention to legs, but away from hips and midsection. Wear belts right at the waist, but no lower, and avoid jeans with faded areas, which can emphasize hips.

love your body

loving what you see

Q **I'm really insecure about my weight. For as long as I can remember, all my friends have been wearing at least a size—if not more—smaller than me, and when I hang out with them, I usually feel like the group blimp. If that's not bad enough, no boy I've ever liked has asked me out. What can I do to lose weight and get the guys I like to like me too?**

A It sounds to us like the most important thing going on here may not be your weight, but your self-esteem. If you're clocking in at a size or two more than your friends who you see as "normal," chances are you're not as large as you think you are. Don't worry, you're not alone. It seems like these days everyone's obsessed with body image. If you obsess over it, and talk about it all the time, this is probably what's going on with you. But keep in mind: When girls constantly complain about their appearance, it makes guys crazy. No guy wants to go out with a girl who has to be told every 10 seconds that her butt isn't too big. It's okay to want to take off a few pounds, but always be comfortable in the skin you're in. Lack of confidence is more of a turnoff than a few extra pounds. Remember: Before others can truly love you, you have to accept yourself for who you are.

Q: I'm overweight, and I have low self-esteem and hardly any confidence. Can you help me with a makeover?

A: Sure, we can talk about a makeover, but the truth is, we should be talking about an inner makeover first. We hear from a lot of girls who lose lots of weight because they think they'll like themselves more. But then they just keep trying to lose more and more because they still don't feel good enough. That's because self-esteem is much more mental than physical, and it's important to be aware of that.

Now, on to your plan! First, ask a doctor if your weight is actually healthy (lots of girls think they're overweight, but they really aren't). If it isn't, work with her or a nutritionist she recommends to put together a workout and diet plan that will help you get to a healthy weight.

Next: confidence and self-esteem. How can you build them up? By doing things that make it very clear to you that you're a lot more than what you look like. Do things you'll be proud of—in school, in your community. If you're proud of yourself in other ways, you'll be a lot more forgiving of your body for not being "perfect." You'll see yourself and be able to show the world that you're not just "the overweight girl in math class." You're the tennis player, the amazing violinist, the talented painter. Everyone's got something they do very, very well. Try a bunch of things and find yours. We truly believe that once you see how powerful you really are, you'll feel better about yourself as a whole.

love your body

Q: I'm repulsed by what I see in the mirror. Just once I want to be able to say, "I look good!"

A: Being pretty (even looking hot) starts on the inside. We know that sounds like the annoying stuff moms say, but it's the truth. And beauty does not come in one form only. At some schools, you have to look a certain way to be considered pretty. If everyone is tan and blond at your school, you might be surprised when you get a ton of compliments on your gorgeous black hair once you go away to college! You need to see your beauty to appreciate being beautiful (which, P.S., you are!). So you're not cookie-cutter—that's a good thing! It means you're unique. Look at your eyes. Your hair. Your mouth. What do you like about yourself? And not just about your face but about you? The way you treat people? The way you play the trumpet? It'll take work, but you'll need to retrain that voice inside your head to say nice things instead of the horrible stuff you just wrote. There are so many people who have had plastic surgery to change themselves into what they thought would be pretty—and they still weren't happy. That feeling comes from inside. We're all beautiful—some of us just don't realize it. But you're going to start today, right?

Q: There hasn't been much going on in my life lately since my boyfriend broke up with me, and the only thing I seem to be fixating on is my ever-growing waistline. I'm actually starting to feel really down about myself over it.

A: Breakups are hard, especially when they're not on your terms. The important thing is to stop feeling sorry for yourself—what you need is a little self TLC. Here's a way to take the focus off of being negative about your body, and being positive for your soul. Before you go to bed, jot down one upside of your day. Focusing on the positive, no matter how miniscule, will make a crappy day seem sweeter. Plus, reading old entries and seeing how far you've come can help you through a rough patch. Once you get a handle on the inside, make positive strides for your outer self. What are some quick confidence boosters? Find your perfect red lipstick. Red lips light up your whole face and make you feel fabulous. Get a part-time job and open a savings account. Slipping a few bucks into the bank each month makes you feel super independent. (Think of how amazing you'll feel when you don't have to ask your mom when you want a new pair of jeans!) Disagree out loud or in writing. Your opinions are as important as anyone else's—so express them! All of these things will make you feel better about yourself. And soon that silly ex-boyfriend will be a distant memory.

love your body

CG! TIP: Put your head in a happy place every day by surrounding yourself with things that say, "I'm fabulous"—like pictures of you with your friends or awards.

Q **Will I ever lose weight? People have told me I'd be a knockout if I lost weight, and I want to lose it because I'm sure it will make me feel better and more outgoing. But I just can't get motivated to do it. Help!**

A Yes, you can lose weight. But your reluctance to do so sounds like there's more going on here. You may be afraid to lose the weight—that the extra pounds are like a cushion between you and the world, a way to avoid having to be a part of things. You need to retrain yourself. What we recommend is that once a week, challenge yourself to do something that's not your norm, like sitting with different people at lunch. Knowing you can overcome challenges—even small ones!—increases your confidence in everything you do, and it will give you the confidence you need to start losing weight. Still insecure about doing it on your own? Why not find a mentor to help you with your diet and exercise? She could be an aunt or a teacher or even one of your mother's friends. Whatever you choose, you have to make a deal with yourself to make an effort; only *you* can change your life. And you can do it as soon as you let yourself!

mean girls

Q In my school, the girls are always comparing themselves to each other. It gets especially bad at prom time, because everyone's dieting to fit into their dresses. Sometimes I just pray, "God, if you can't make me thin, please make everyone else fat." How am I going to get through this?

A Bad body image is like a virus: It's easy to catch. But if you've caught a case of bad body image from a friend, you can reverse it easily enough. To get out of the bad mind-set, think about someone you really admire (someone you actually know, as opposed to a famous person). What do you like about her—and don't say that she's skinny. Totally forget what she looks like. Maybe it's her athletic ability or sense of humor, or how she treats you. If you focus on qualities like these, instead of thinking it all has to do with looks, you'll quickly learn what you really value in others—and yourself. Next, cultivate friendships that are based on helping each other feel strong. Relay positive messages to friends and you can even create a deeper bond with them.

love your body

Q: My friends tell me I'm fat. I can't help but think they're right. What should I do?

A: First and foremost: Make new friends. You need to be around people who empower you, not ones who make you feel bad about yourself. This is not as hard as you may think. In school, there may be people outside your group you'd like to know a little better. This is your chance to consciously choose your friends. So get a pencil and paper and write down those things your current girl group isn't giving you. (You may be surprised how little they are giving you—aside from terrible self-esteem!) You don't have to only make friends with people in your school. Maybe there's a bookstore you like to hang out in, or maybe you have an after-school job where there are interesting people for you to hang out with. True, it can feel weird talking to people you don't know. But making friends is like getting new shoes: You try on a lot, take a few home, and then eventually you know what you like to go with every day!

jerky boys

Q **I wish I could lose weight. I feel ugly and like no one will ever want to date me. My ex-boyfriend told me I was fat and that no one would want me after we broke up. I would like to lose all this weight—so he'll wish he still had me.**

A You know what we think? You're holding on to that lousy ex-boyfriend by actually becoming the overweight girl he always said you were. When you get rid of his bad energy, you will be able to get rid of the weight. Gather everything he ever gave you and make a list of all the mean things he said. Then throw them out or put them in a box and throw it away. As you do, say, "The weight is my ex." When your mind makes that connection, your body will too. Once you've cleared out the negative energy, fill that space with images of who you want to be. At first, you might imagine the kind of girl your ex would come crawling back to. But soon you'll stop thinking about what he likes and start being true to yourself. He may want you back, but by then, you won't want to be with a loser like him.

love your body

Q **This guy at school always calls me "fat" and "ugly." I try not to let it get to me, but who likes being picked on, right? Other girls are chunkier, but he says nothing to them. Why does he pick on me?**

A Here's the truth: Anyone who dogs on someone for the way they look is totally lame. You can only feel bad for the guy—he clearly has low self-esteem. Think about it: If he felt so great, would he need to be rude? Do you think someone on top of their game needs to put people down? Why bother?! The only people who do are people who feel bad about themselves or are hurting inside. The way they express these negative feelings is by lashing out at others—and making them feel bad. But you're too smart for that! We bet you're really good at something. Maybe you get good grades, or have the kind of family that this guy wishes he had. He's envious of something, which is why you're his target. Boohoo for him! Here's your plan: Just laugh yourself into your soon-to-be super-empowered, happy life. We know, it's easier to say this than to do it, but still: Ignore him! The more he gets under your skin, the more he tricks himself into thinking he's a big man. Just keep going for your goals, keep being a nice person—and know that you are so freaking special, talented, gorgeous (everything!) that you made some poor fool so jealous, he couldn't even act human. Impressive!

parent trap

Q I remember my mom being concerned about my weight from a really early age, even though I wasn't overweight. At dinner, she'd give a big portion to my father, a medium portion to herself, and the smallest potion to me. She didn't say a word, but I knew what she was thinking: She wanted me to be thin. I'm 19 now, and whenever I look in the mirror, I still feel that judgment. What can I do?

A Without meaning to, it looks like your mom taught you to feel bad about your body. But just because an idea comes from your parents doesn't mean it's true. Maybe it's not always directed at you—maybe your dad is constantly telling your sister to go on a diet, or your mom's had plastic surgery 3 times—and she's only 40. Things like that can really affect—or should we say, infect—your own idea of beautiful, as you're seeing now. Don't worry: You can change it. Try to identify these negative messages from your parents and see if they really hold up. Ask your mom and dad how they feel about their own bodies, and what their parents told them about health and eating and weight. It's possible that they don't even

love your body

realize what they were doing. The most important thing you need to be able to do is to put those comments in their proper place; don't internalize them and feel bad about yourself. Ever!

Q **My mom and dad always belittle my achievements. I get good grades, but they're always harping on my looks. They think I'm overweight, and they remind me about it all the time. I'm not as thin as my sister, but I'm in the healthy range. That's not enough for them, though. How can I get them to see me as worthwhile?**

A Here's the thing about getting people to think you're worthwhile: You have to believe you're worthy, not look to other people to confirm you are. It's time to shift your mind-set so that you're succeeding for you. That way, you'll feel the kind of respect you've been craving from others, including your parents. You won't care as much about whether you get approval from others because you'll feel it where it counts: inside. Which is not to say you should put your hurt feelings on a back shelf. The next time you're alone with your mom, say, "I've been upset because I can't make you happy. No matter how well I do in school, all you seem to see is my weight. How can I make you proud of me?" Your mom might be surprised and apologize and tell you why she acts the way she does, or she might—and prepare yourself—get defensive and tell you she "doesn't want to hear it." In any case, you'll feel better putting your feelings out there.

CG! TIP: Your family's eating habits can affect your health, so take a step back and make sure those habits are good ones!

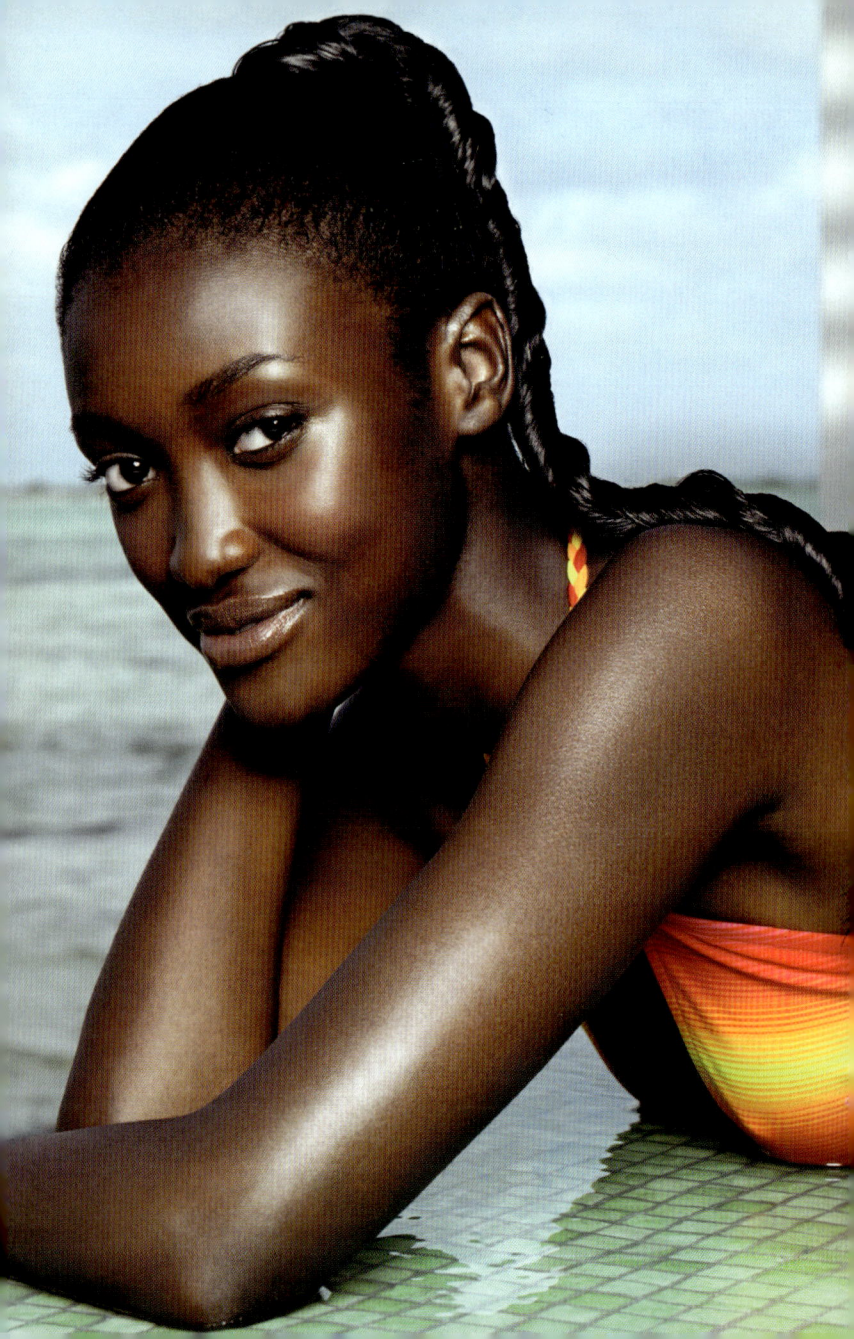

chapter 4

weighty issues

A healthy diet, regular exercise, and good self-esteem are the cornerstones of looking—and feeling—great. But sometimes our fixations to look and feel a certain way can turn destructive and, instead of becoming healthier, they can make us sick—in our bodies and our minds. Do any of these questions from your fellow CosmoGIRL!s in this chapter sound like you? If they do, you may want to talk to someone about it. You owe it to yourself, CG!

> If you're down and don't know where to turn, call The Renfrew Center Foundation at 1-877-367-3383. Don't worry, it will be confidential and it could change your life.

weighty issues

food obsession

Q **I eat when I'm bored, angry, depressed, or sad, and I've noticed that I've been gaining a lot of weight lately because of it. But I can't seem to help myself. What should I do?**

A We recommend that you find other ways to keep yourself busy. Right away! There are many things you could be doing instead of dipping into the cookie jar when you're bored. The trick is to be creative—keep yourself interested! Here are a few suggestions— try some and see if they spark any more bright ideas. How about one of the needle arts—like knitting or crochet. These require the use of both hands, and you won't want to get your creation sticky, saucy, or otherwise messy with food—not after you worked so hard on it! You could also turn your energies to growing something. Visit a nursery to find out what plants grow best in your area, then plant seeds. You could also sign up for lessons. Have you always wanted to learn to play the piano? That takes focus, concentration—and both hands. You could look into doing something nice for others—see about starting a (snack-free) story hour at your library. Of course, the best idea is doing something physical—like a karate class. You'll keep yourself out of the fridge—and chop away calories while you're at it. Hi-yah!

Q **Lately, whether or not I eat is like a contest—between me and food. I'm not sure when this started, but it doesn't feel very healthy. Why is this happening to me—and how can I stop it?**

A The most messed-up relationship some of us will ever have won't be with a person, but with food! How does a basic necessity become such a twisted obsession? Basically, from the time we're babies, food is used to soothe us—a bottle calms us down when we cry, etc. In your situation, it doesn't seem like it's totally about the food, but more like there's something else that feels out of control in your life. Maybe you're floundering in school or there's trouble at home? Whatever might be causing this fixation, we urge you to look into it and try to get help right away. Make an appointment with your guidance counselor or a therapist—seek the advice of a responsible adult who can assist you in grappling with your other problems and help you get your head straight. Whether or not you eat will become more serious the longer you do this dance with yourself, but if you get to the root of the real problem, and then tackle and overcome it, we feel like you'll win your contest with food.

weighty issues

Q **Until around 3:30 PM, just looking at food makes me want to puke, so I usually skip breakfast and lunch. But then I get so hungry that I pig out. How can I stop?**

A Feeling sick at the sight of food is definitely not a good thing. But there might be a simple reason—and remedy. Could it be that you just don't like the food you're faced with in the morning and at lunchtime? If breakfast means a greasy plate of fried eggs and bacon, and your stomach can't handle heavy food first thing, that can make you queasy. Even the sight of milk makes many people uneasy. The same goes for lunch: Cafeteria food isn't exactly known for winning awards for culinary excellence! But by not fueling your body for the most active parts of the day, you're forcing your brain to strain to concentrate. That causes your muscles to become sluggish and less responsive. Then when you finally do eat, your body is forced to use the little energy it does have for digestion. That draws blood away from your brain and extremities, causing you to feel more sluggish and maybe a bit woozy. Here are some suggestions:

- Instead of starving yourself, talk to your parents about fixing meals that include foods you'll look forward to eating. You might find that in the morning and early afternoon, you still need to eat lighter foods like breakfast bars, yogurt, pretzels, or a smoothie.
- It's okay to eat several mini-meals during the day. Bring snacks with you to eat when the mood strikes during school. By eating little meals throughout the day, you'll be much less likely to overeat after school.

But if none of this helps, and you still can't bear to put anything in your mouth before mid-afternoon and then pig out later in the day, you might have a problem called binge-eating disorder, which isn't really about food—it's about having control. Binge eaters use food to distract themselves from emotional problems, so to eat healthfully again, they need to deal with those issues with the help of a specialist trained in eating disorders. If it goes untreated, it can lead to high blood pressure, heart disease, and diabetes. If you think this might be the problem, check out the National Eating Disorders Association at nationaleatingdisorders.org, or call 800-931-2237 for more information.

weighty issues

reality check

Q My mother and my friends tell me that I'm obese, but I tell them that I just like to eat. I'm only 16 years old. I want to enjoy my life now, and I'll diet when I get to college and when I'm older. What's wrong with that?

A We're sorry to say, but there are many things wrong with that. First of all, being overweight at any time in your life can be potentially dangerous. And if it's true what your mom and friends are saying about you being obese, there are many health risks associated with that.

- You can develop joint problems in your ankles and hips—and you could even risk dislocating your hips. Back pain is also common when you carry too much extra weight.
- Breathing, which should be as effortless as, well, breathing, also becomes a problem when you're obese. On top of that, you also risk sleep apnea, which causes snoring and briefly stops you from breathing when you sleep—which can lead to heart disease later in life.

- You can develop ovarian cysts, acne, male-pattern hair growth—like hair on your chin and chest—as well as irregular periods and even infertility.
- There's also a chance of developing diabetes, which brings with it a whole slew of problems, including fatigue, damage to your circulation, and eventually high blood pressure. In severe cases of diabetes, you can become blind, and if your circulation to your limbs gets so bad, you run the risk of hand and foot amputation.
- And don't forget about your liver! Fat accumulation in the liver can lead to liver damage and possible liver failure—and you may even need a transplant.

So...we do feel strongly that it's better for you to start losing some weight now. See your doctor, who can help you get started on a healthy weight-loss plan where you can still enjoy eating. Because liking to eat is a healthy thing.

weighty issues

Q: Is being overweight as a teenager really a health risk—or isn't it much later in life when it becomes a problem?

A: If you're overweight, you absolutely have to take action now, and not wait until you're older to worry about the risks. In fact, there's a 7-percent chance that overweight teens will remain overweight as adults—putting them at risk for heart disease, high blood pressure, and more. How can you make sure you're not one of them? Limit TV watching, videogame playing, and computer use to two hours a day. Then get up and move. Also, choose drinks that don't have tons of sugar, salt, carbonation, chemicals, or calories—like water or skim milk. Finally, watch portion sizes: Study labels to find out what the real serving size is. (One cup is about a handful, not a plateful!)

CG! TIP: Taking 10 slow, deep breaths in through your nose and out through your mouth can relax your whole body. Try it the next time you feel stressed or nervous.

smoking away the pounds

Q: I started smoking to keep my weight down, and it's really worked. I don't see the harm of smoking when I'm young. Don't I have to smoke for years before it affects my health?

A: Don't believe that smoking keeps you thin. When you smoke, you don't eat, and that's why you lose weight. But there are plenty of less harmful ways to keep your eating under control. It doesn't matter how old you are: Smoking will kill you. You have to quit right away. In the United States alone, 38,000 people die each year from diseases caused by secondhand smoke. Also, 57 percent more women will die of lung cancer than of breast cancer this year. And why is it never a good time to start? Seventh graders who smoke are 21 percent more likely to go on to smoke pot and 36 times more likely to do hard drugs. On top of that, smoking burns your throat, it makes your clothes and hair smell bad, and it can even turn your fingers yellow. What's cool about that? To get help quitting, call the American Cancer Society at 800-ACS-2345, or head to trytostop.org.

weighty issues

Q: I started smoking because all the skinny girls I knew smoked cigarettes. And now I can't stop. What should I do?

A It may be hard to kick the habit, but you've already taken a very important step—you've decided you have to give it up! Good for you! If quitting cold turkey seems like it will be too hard to do, don't worry. There are many other options. Consider joining a cessation program. The support of others helps lots of people kick the habit. Call the American Cancer Society at 800-ACS-2345 to find programs in your area. You could also try nicotine replacements, which help control your urge for nicotine by giving you progressively smaller doses. Available at drugstores and by prescription, they come in many forms—gum, the patch, and lozenges. Doctors can also prescribe nicotine-free bupropion (Zyban) to smokers (even teens) to help control their urge to light up. Get more information at tobaccofree.com. Some former smokers have benefited from alternative techniques, like hypnosis and acupuncture, but there is no scientific proof that these work.

Q: I am overweight and have tried unsuccessfully for years to lose weight. Should I consider gastric bypass surgery?

A: Gastric bypass surgery is a controversial procedure that reduces the size of your stomach from a football to an egg. Risks include nutritional deficiencies like anemia and osteoporosis, malnutrition, and gallstones. For these reasons especially, not everyone is given the option to have gastric bypass surgery. Talk to your doctor to see if you're a viable candidate. For the most part, candidates for this type of surgery must have a Body Mass Index-for-age in the ninety-fifth percentile and a life-threatening obesity-related health problem like diabetes, severe sleep apnea, or heart disease. If you are eligible for the surgery, however, know what you're getting into. Head to asbs.org for more information.

index

Apples, benefits of, 57
Asian wraps, 20

Bloating, 56
Breakfast, 14–18
    for dinner, 25
    fatigue after eating, 16, 17
    healthy, suggestions,
      16–18
    low-fat options, 18
    not liking, 15
    skipping, 14
    working up to eating, 15
Butt
    drawing attention away
      from, 99
    toning, 76

Chicken dinner, 68
Chicken wrap, 67
Christmas, eating during, 24
Clothes
    drawing attention away
      from hips, 99
    fit of, to track weight
      consistency, 97
    fitting/choosing jeans,
      98, 99
    tops for top-heavy girls, 99
    for working out, 83
Coffee
    benefits of, 36, 38
    calorie content, 36, 37
    drawbacks of, 38
    warm vs. iced, 37

Dancing, 87
Dessert, 33–35
    fondue dip, 35
    ice cream alternative, 34
    mixed-berry trifle, 33
Dieting dilemmas, 69–71
Diet myths, 50–52
Digestive problems, 57
Dining out, 25–30
    choosing between items,
      27, 30
    eating at home vs., 25
    fast-food suggestions,
      28–29
    healthy menu selections,
      26
    hunger after, 29
    portion control and, 41,
      70–71
Dinner
    with family, 25
    at home vs. dining out, 25
Dip, low-fat, 21
Drinks, 36–40. *See also*
    Coffee; Smoothies
    bottled vs. tap water, 40
    comparison of, 39–40
    energy drinks vs.
      chocolate milk, 39
    flavored vs. plain water, 40
    water intake
      requirements, 38

Eating disorders resources,
    117
Eating out. *See* Dining out

Exercising. *See* Working out

Fake Banana Cream Pie, 48–49
Fat. *See also* Low-fat ideas
 fast food and, 28
 importance of, in diet, 18
 in reduced-fat muffin, 27
 unhealthy (trans/hydrogenated), 27
Fatigue, after breakfast, 16, 17
Fondue dip, 35
Food labels, 43, 53
Food obsessions, 114–117
Fruit salsa with pita chips, 22

Gastric bypass surgery, 123

Habits, healthy, 12–13, 44–46
Healthy diet, 10–71. *See also* Snacks
 apples and, 57
 breakfast tips, 14–18
 desserts, 33–35
 dieting dilemmas, 69–71
 diet myths, 50–52
 dining out, 25–30
 drinks, 36–40. *See also* Coffee; Smoothies
 fast healthy food, 66–68
 habits for, 12–13, 44–46
 metabolism and, 31–32
 minerals and, 54–55, 69
 party tricks, 19–23
 portion control, 41–43, 45, 70–71
 speed of eating, 46
 varying diet, 55
 vegetarianism and, 54–55, 58–65
 weight issues and. *See* Losing weight; Weight
Holiday eating, 24
Hydrating yourself, 38

Jeans, fitting/choosing, 98, 99

Losing weight. *See also* Weight
 choice for, 104–105
 clothes fitting and, 97
 dieting dilemmas, 69–71
 diet myths, 50–52
 diet plans, 52
 fear of, 104
 gastric bypass surgery for, 123
 metabolism and, 31–32
 not weighing yourself and, 97
 portion control and, 41–43, 45, 70–71
 self-esteem/confidence and, 100–108, 109–110
 skipping breakfast and, 14
 skipping meals and, 14, 51
 smoking for, 121–122
 vegetarianism and, 60

index

Loving your body, 94–111. See also Losing weight; Weight
  choosing clothes and. See Clothes
  looking beyond physical things, 105–106
  mean peers and, 105–106
  not comparing yourself and, 96, 105–106
  poor parental feedback and, 109–111
  self-esteem/confidence and, 100–108, 109–110
Low-fat ideas
  breakfast foods, 18
  dips, 21
  holiday foods, 24
  keeping some fat in diet, 18
  Tex-Mex food, 23

Metabolism, 31–32
Minerals, 54–55, 69
Mixed-berry trifle, 33

Overweight/obesity risks, 118–120. See also Losing weight; Weight

Parental feedback, poor, 109–111
Parties, 19–23
  healthy snack ideas, 20–22
  holiday eating, 24
  low-fat dips, 21
  not overeating at, 19
  tasty low-fat Tex-Mex food, 23
Pasta, portions, 41
Pie, 48–49
Portion control, 41–43, 45, 70–71
Protein
  increasing, 29
  lack of, indicators, 16, 29
  vegetarianism and, 62, 64

Restaurants. See Dining out
Running, 82–84, 92

Self-esteem/confidence, weight and, 100–108, 109–110
Shoes, for working out, 84
Skipping meals, 12, 14, 51
Sleeping, weight gain and, 69
Smoking, 121–122
Smoothies
  recipes, 16, 17, 18
  sugar content, 27
Snacks, 47–49
  healthy suggestions, 20–22
  before meals, 48–49
  portion sizes, 42
  reducing junk food, 47
  satisfying, not greasy/salty, 22
Stomach
  puffy, 56
  working out abs, 74–75
Strawberry-yogurt parfait, 34

Stretching, 93
Sugar
    fatigue after eating, 16
    in fruit, 27

Tex-Mex food, 23
Tuna salad whole-wheat pita, 66
TV, eating while watching, 44

Vegetarian facts/fiction, 54–55, 58–65
Vitamins and minerals, 54–55, 65, 69

Walking, 81, 86
Water
    bottled vs. tap, 40
    flavored vs. plain, 40
    intake requirements, 38
Weight, 112–123. *See also* Losing weight
    food obsessions and, 114–117
    jeans fitting and, 98, 99
    mean peers and, 105–106
    muscle vs. fat, 97
    not comparing yourself with others, 96, 105–106
    overweight/obesity risks, 118–120
    people belittling you about, 105–111
    self-esteem/confidence and, 100–108, 109–110

Working out, 72–93
    abs, 74–75
    aches and pains from, 92–93
    avoiding injury, 93
    benefits of, 77, 91
    for bikini fit, 88
    cheerleading and, 89
    clothing for, 83
    cooling down after, 90
    dancing, 87
    listening to music while, 90
    making it fun, 85–91
    motivation for, 78, 85, 86
    running, 82–84, 92
    schedules/routines, 77–81
    shoes for, 84
    stretching and, 93
    toning butt, 76
    walking, 81, 86
    weight substitutes, 91

Also available:

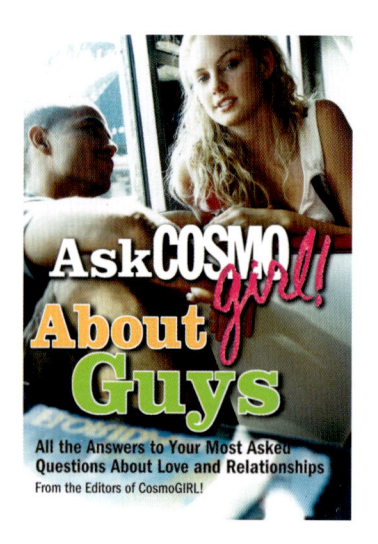

Ask COSMOgirl! About Guys
All the Answers to Your Most Asked Questions About Love and Relationships
From the Editors of CosmoGIRL!

978-1-58816-485-8
$5.95/ $7.95 Can.

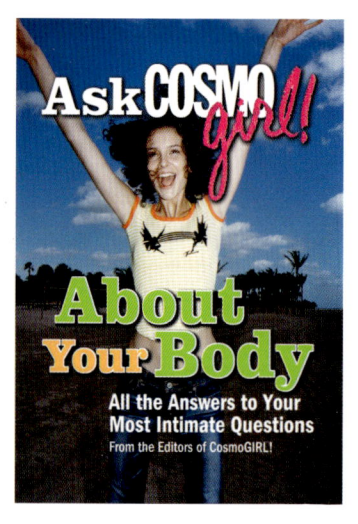

Ask COSMOgirl! About Your Body
All the Answers to Your Most Intimate Questions
From the Editors of CosmoGIRL!

978-1-58816-486-5
$5.95/ $7.95 Can.